Unravelling Workplace Culture in Healthcare

Lauren Philp-von Woyna

Unravelling Workplace Culture in Healthcare

A Guide for Practitioners to Explore, Understand and Change

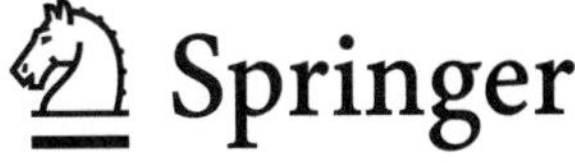 Springer

Lauren Philp-von Woyna
Department of Nursing and Midwifery
University of Birmingham
Birmingham, UK

ISBN 978-3-032-11770-0   ISBN 978-3-032-11771-7   (eBook)
https://doi.org/10.1007/978-3-032-11771-7

This Springer imprint is published by the registered company Springer Nature Switzerland AG
The registered company address is: Gewerbestrasse 11, 6330 Cham, Switzerland

If disposing of this product, please recycle the paper.

*For my six beautiful children, Annabel,
Amaris, Arthur, Ethan, Aaron, Noah.*

Preface

When my fifth child was born, I was an experienced midwife and midwifery teacher. I was a passionate, keen teacher and I prioritised teaching students about the importance of compassionate care while endeavouring to produce the best midwives who would influence the profession globally. However, I never anticipated that I would personally suffer at the hands of those I taught.

I had four children already, and I felt confident about having my fifth child assuming I would be treated with respect. I knew my rights, my choices and what to look for to make sure me and my baby were well. Despite my knowledge, I experienced a traumatic birth that lacked informed consent, compassion and kindness. My son has a significant, lifelong disability and while I can't say for certain it was due to the substandard care I received, it led me to question and feel ashamed of my profession as a midwife. I found myself asking why, and how the people I had personally invested in through education could ignore my concerns, display such a lack compassion and fail to recognise a problem. I felt angry and disappointed at the state of maternity care in the UK. It prompted me to think about why people act the way they do in healthcare, sometimes when they seem to know the evidence base, and I questioned why my power and voice changed when I became a labouring mother instead of a senior midwife and midwifery teacher. What are the powerful, often unspoken undercurrents of influence that cause individuals and groups to act in ways that cause harm or do not stop harm? It may not even be intentional, but somehow it has become acceptable.

It is painful to see that UK national reports into maternity care continue to report the same issues I have personally experienced. Women are not being listened to when receiving maternity care [1], there is continued poor team working, poor decision making, inability to recognise the severity of problems and generally a poor workplace culture that continues to lead to poor outcomes for mothers and babies [2]. Like many women before me and many women since my experience, concerns raised by patients or team members in healthcare are often dismissed and shutdown. While much of my own experience can be attributed to the individuals providing care, those individuals were also part of a team on the ward, a wider organisation and a global profession. All of the social and professional layers, identities and powers associated with being a midwife influence the way an individual midwife behaves. This is not only true for midwives but also for other health professionals. The layers of social and culture-based factors affect their every day care provided, and at times, these different layers might enable poor healthcare practice to continue.

Writing this book is both difficult and satisfying. It is difficult because addressing issues of workplace culture is enormously complex, but it is satisfying because I hope it will inspire and enable positive culture-based change in healthcare. I have devoted my doctoral studies to understanding the socio-cultural factors that influence learning and idea sharing behaviour in the healthcare context, and this book delves into what I discovered listening to those who provide care as connected to wider theory and literature.

Birmingham, UK   Lauren Philp-von Woyna

References

1. All-Party Parliamentary Group. Birth trauma: listen to mums – ending the postcode lottery on perinatal care [Internet]. London: UK Parliament; 2024. Available from: https://www.theo-clarke.org.uk/sites/www.theo-clarke.org.uk/files/2024-05/Birth%20Trauma%20Inquiry%20Report%20for%20Publication_May13_2024.pdf.
2. Department of Health and Social Care. Final report of the Ockenden review: findings, conclusions and essential actions from the independent review of maternity services at the Shrewsbury and Telford Hospital NHS Trust [Internet]. London: GOV.UK; 2022. Available from: https://www.gov.uk/government/publications/final-report-of-the-ockenden-review.

Acknowledgements

This book is written with special thanks to the people who have encouraged and helped me shape the work; Dr Ruth Hudson, Professor Gillian Forrester, Professor Caroline Bradbury-Jones and everyone at the University of Birmingham writing group.

About the Book

Workplace culture is about how people work together, what they value and the behaviours and practices they foster, encourage and build or do not. Culture is defined as the ideas, customs and social behaviour of a particular people or society [1]. It is also defined as the traditional behaviour which has been developed and is successively learned by each generation. The *culture* of groups includes specific established attitudes, values, beliefs and practices which are exhibited within the group, and which have been shown to affect the health and wellbeing of employees, the working environment and the quality and safety of healthcare provided [1, 2]. The culture of healthcare groups might allow or even enable poor practice that negatively affects both patients and staff [2]. Such behaviours might include ignoring concerns raised by individuals or allowing anti-social behaviours like bullying to continue that lead to psychological harm.

Workplace culture in healthcare matters because a positive group culture can improve safety, wellbeing and response to increasing demands and challenges in healthcare. Major challenges in today's healthcare include demands to meet the changing healthcare needs of older and more complex patients (whose needs are often unmet), long-term underinvestment/underfunding in healthcare and its consequences, persistent staff shortages, staff burnout and public dissatisfaction [3]. Working in high-pressure, under-resourced teams providing healthcare can alter how we behave towards each other and how effectively we work together. Factors such as high-stress levels, lack of social support, conflicts, unfair treatment, demanding workload, poor communication, lack of support from authority figures, and a loss of sense of control and autonomy contribute towards increasing likelihood of staff burnout [4]. Many of these factors can be influenced locally, at the individual level, while other factors are more closely related to organisational-level and/or workplace leadership.

Local social behaviour (how we interact with each other, about each other and work together as a team) is widely reported as problematic in healthcare. A recent report documented 87 accounts of bullying in maternity settings as described by 37 newly qualified midwives and 50 student midwives [5] and local social-based problems such as negative gossip in healthcare [6] and assigning blame to each other when problems arise are commonly reported [7]. These behaviours are damaging to individual wellbeing and teamworking [7].

Negative behaviour issues such as bullying, blame and negative gossip raise crucial social questions such as why do people *join in*, stand by or enable these kinds of poor workplace behaviour. What are the barriers that individuals and organisations face in addressing poor social behaviour? And what can be done to recognise and change the ways healthcare professionals and organisations work together?

Everyday healthcare practice happens in and is influenced by *socio-cultural factors* because healthcare professionals work together in a social and cultural context to provide care. Socio-cultural factors are defined as the interactions between the individual, the social community and the broader cultural environment [8]. Studying the workplace culture from a socio-cultural perspective requires examination of how the person in context acts, including what motivates them, what ideas for innovation and improvement they share and act upon, what goals they want to achieve and the meaning they give to their own work [9]. Socio-cultural theory suggests that people are constrained or afforded possibilities in their work by the workplace environment or their position and by culture-based norms (usual ways of working) of the group [9]. This may seem like a complex theory with many layers, but essentially socio-cultural theory claims that individuals act in ways that are influenced by their social connections, workplace culture and wider culture. This impacts whether they feel they are able to make valuable contributions at work (their perception of power and value), able to share their ideas and able to act upon them to improve healthcare (their confidence in their own ability to bring positive change to healthcare). In current literature, there is limited focus given to socio-cultural factors influencing everyday healthcare practice, including how it shapes workplace culture, organisational structures, workplace hierarchy and impacts new ideas, innovations and improvements, as well as individual wellbeing and sense of purpose in work.

This book is an essential read for any health professional (and related staff) because problematic workplace culture is an increasingly reported issue in national and international health-related investigations and reviews. It is essential to understand that workplace culture is partly a manifestation of the system pressures, under-resourcing and underfunding of health services, but also partly down to the individuals working within healthcare (how they communicate with each other, work together and what they allow to happen around them). Every healthcare worker holds the power to decide what practices (behaviours, values, attitudes) they will allow to happen where they work and what practices they will not tolerate. Therefore, the individual healthcare worker is a hugely powerful agent in changing workplace culture. Changing workplace culture in healthcare requires a multi-level approach: firstly, system level changes are needed, and secondly, individual/local level changes are needed. From a socio-cultural perspective, workplace culture-based issues in healthcare can be traced back to both system issues *and* individual/local issues. Both of these need to be addressed to change workplace culture-based issues.

An example that frames the focus of this book well and illustrates how system-level and individual/local-level socio-cultural factors come together can be understood through everyday practice in primary care. In the UK, individuals make an appointment to see their General Practitioner (GP) doctor by telephoning the GP practice. This encounter can differ depending on the person's social factors and the workplace culture of the GP practice. If the individual lives in an area with an excessive backlog and shortage of GP appointments, their social position (which includes where they live) might impact their ability to *access* a GP. It is not uncommon for access to GP appointments to be problematic in some geographical areas in the UK. During April 2024, 1.6 million people had waited longer than a month to have a GP appointment in the UK [10], with the UK's Office for National Statistics (ONS) reporting that 33% of patients found it difficult or very difficult to contact their GP [11].

Varied access to a timely GP service contributes towards inequalities and impacts people living in areas of higher deprivation more often. Evidence suggests that GPs working in areas that are under-resourced experience *a different workplace culture* compared to those in better-resourced areas. Socio-cultural factors and theory can help to explain how work pressures can directly influence workplace culture, team-working and wellbeing. For example, when backlogs for booking GP appointments occur, it impacts the GPs and other staff working in those areas influencing social behaviours and what it feels like to work there. Under-resourced GPs face both unsustainable and insurmountable workloads as well as increased complaints and inability to provide the care they want to give [10]. Nearly 100,000 complaints were made about GP services during the year 2021/2022 [12]. The most common reasons for complaints included communication issues (14%), errors in care provided (13%) and poor staff attitude, values or behaviour (13%) [12]. Two of the top three reasons for complaints relate to social (interaction and communication) and culture-based factors (attitude, norms, values and behaviour). This finding is not unique to GP services but is common across multiple national healthcare inquiries and reports [13–16]. It illustrates that system-level decisions and culture, impact adequate resourcing of health services which subsequently alters what it is like at the individual, local and social level to work in healthcare. The social-culture (socio-cultural) environment influences individual wellbeing, ability to work as a team and patient safety. It is a topic which has inspired my own research and informs the foundation for this book because when incidents or errors happen in healthcare, I believe an aspect of understanding those issues/errors needs to be understood as a manifestation of socio-cultural issues, both at the system level and local level, as intertwined and inseparable. Socio-cultural perspectives of workplace culture aid understanding about why and how some workplace culture-based problems develop and can persist and how ideas to change problematic culture can be supported to flourish.

This book takes you through the multiple layers of different social and culture-based factors that influence individual health professional behaviour, the generation of ideas and the courage and confidence to act on ideas to improve healthcare workplace culture. The aim is to ensure every healthcare worker has a better understanding about what enables or constrains the type of workplace they want to find themselves leading or working within.

My doctoral research has formed the understanding and foundation of topics covered in this book. Each chapter is focussed on an area of findings from my research as linked to current healthcare challenges and improvement ideas. The book intends to engage you throughout, with reflective tasks, research extracts, theoretical and applied examples and anecdotes. Each chapter can be read in isolation; however, you will gain a better understanding about how workplace culture-based issues are intertwined by reading the text in full.

References

1. Simpson D, Hamilton S, McSherry R, McIntosh R. Measuring and assessing healthcare organisational culture in England's National Health Service: a snapshot of current tools and tool use. Healthcare (Basel). 2019;7(4):127. https://doi.org/10.3390/healthcare7040127. PMID: 31683839; PMCID: PMC6955975.
2. Philp-Von Woyna L. A multi-case study to understand the ways in which sociocultural factors influence everyday creative contributions in healthcare and higher education by student midwives. Doctoral thesis. Staffordshire: Staffordshire University; 2025. Available from: https://eprints.staffs.ac.uk/8884/.
3. Dunn P, Ewbank L, Alderwick H. Nine major challenges facing health and care in England. London: The Health Foundation; 2023. Available from: https://www.health.org.uk/reports-and-analysis/briefings/nine-major-challenges-facing-health-and-care-in-england.
4. Medina-Dominguez F, Sanchez-Segura MI, de Amescua-Seco A, Dugarte-Peña GL, Villalba Arranz S. Agile Delphi methodology: a case study on how technology impacts burnout syndrome in the post-pandemic era. Front Public Health. 2023;10. https://doi.org/10.3389/fpubh.2022.
5. Burleigh A, Wylam J, Millar B, Gillen P, Webster J, McEwen K, et al. #Saynotobullyinginmidwifery: trigger warning – this report contains frank accounts of bullying behaviours and consequences [ebook]. Amanda Burleigh; 2023. Available from: https://www.amazon.co.uk/dp/1399969005.
6. Georganta K, Panagopoulou E, Montgomery A. Talking behind their backs: negative gossip and burnout in hospitals. Burnout Res. 2014. https://doi.org/10.1016/j.burn.2014.07.003.
7. Radhakrishna S. Culture of blame in the National Health Service; consequences and solutions. Br J Anaesth. 2015;115(5):653–5. Available from: https://www.bjanaesthesia.org.
8. Csíkszentmihályi M. Creativity: flow and the psychology of discovery and invention. New York: Harper Collins; 1996.
9. Glăveanu VP, Hanchett Hanson M, Baer J, Barbot B, Clapp E, Corazza E, et al. Advancing creativity theory and research: a socio-cultural manifesto. J Creat Behav. 2020;54:741–5.
10. The Health Foundation. UK GPs suffering unsustainable workplace pressures [Internet]. London: The Health Foundation; 2023. Available from: https://www.health.org.uk/press-office/press-releases/uk-gps-suffering-unsustainable-workplace-pressures.
11. Office for National Statistics. Experiences of NHS healthcare services in England: July 2025 [Internet]. Newport (UK): ONS; 2025. Available from: https://www.ons.gov.uk/peoplepopulationandcommunity/healthandsocialcare/healthcaresystem/bulletins/experiencesofnhshealthcareservicesinengland/july2025.
12. NHS Digital. Data on written complaints in the NHS, 2021–22 [Internet]. Leeds: NHS Digital; 2022. Available from: https://digital.nhs.uk/data-and-information/publications/statistical/data-on-written-complaints-in-the-nhs/2021-22.
13. Department of Health and Social Care. Final report of the Ockenden review: findings, conclusions and essential actions from the independent review of maternity services at the Shrewsbury and Telford Hospital NHS Trust [Internet]. London: GOV.UK; 2022. Available from: https://www.gov.uk/government/publications/final-report-of-the-ockenden-review.

14. Nursing and Midwifery Council. NMC register leavers' survey: summary 2024 [Internet]. London: NMC; 2024. Available from: https://www.nmc.org.uk.

15. Department of Health and Social Care. Reading the signals: maternity and neonatal services in East Kent – the report of the independent investigation [Internet]. London: GOV.UK; 2022. Available from: https://www.gov.uk/government/publications/maternity-and-neonatal-services-in-east-kent-reading-the-signals-report.

16. All-Party Parliamentary Group on Birth Trauma. Listen to mums: ending the postcode lottery on perinatal care [Internet]. London: UK Parliament; 2024. Available from: https://www.theo-clarke.org.uk/birth-trauma-inquiry.

Contents

About the Author

As a midwife and Associate Professor of Midwifery Education, my doctoral research focussed on the socio-cultural factors that influence idea-sharing (creativity) and learning in healthcare [1]. Creativity-based research, especially relating to healthcare practice or education, is extremely limited, while the benefits of enabling idea-sharing across other subject areas is widely acknowledged and studied. My study focussed on idea-sharing that occurred specifically in the midwifery practice or higher education context and highlighted the promising benefits of motivating and enabling idea-sharing in healthcare for improving care and solving health-related challenges.

Healthcare is highly demanding, unpredictable and ever-changing, and it often requires significant emotional involvement and investment by healthcare workers. There is increasing demand to meet emerging and developing health service needs that require workers and healthcare organisations to be innovative, creatively agile and responsive. Creativity (through the sharing of and acting on new ideas) is imperative for addressing current challenges in healthcare and is also strongly associated with individual healthcare worker psychological wellbeing and patient safety. While existing literature highlights the importance of thinking and acting in new ways, the emergence of idea-sharing is shaped by local sociocultural factors. However, this area remains underexplored, especially within specific contexts such as healthcare practice and education. This matters because understanding factors that motivate, enable or constrain new ways of thinking and working is important for enabling healthcare improvement and innovation.

My research adopted a constructivist, qualitative multi-case study design that explored student midwives perspectives about socio-cultural factors that motivate, enable or constrain new everyday creative ideas and contributions in healthcare [1]. A case study is a methodology aids understanding about phenomena in-depth and within its real-world context, especially where the boundaries between phenomenon and context are not clearly understood [2]. A multi-case study typically examines several individual case studies to analyse similarities across numerous cases. My doctoral multi-case study focussed on answering research questions related to specific contextual conditions which may have influenced idea-sharing and creative contributions (acting on ideas shared) by student midwives. The multi-case study methodology was particularly appropriate because the boundaries related to socio-cultural factors that influence creative ideas in healthcare are not clearly understood.

The intention was to understand how an individual's position, perspective/belief, wider and local policy and micro-politics, social connections and educational opportunities influence their idea-sharing and improvement efforts in healthcare.

Eight participants from an undergraduate midwifery programme were treated as single case studies which were later analysed together in cross-case analysis. Each case provided in-depth detail about idea-sharing and creative action to solve current challenges in healthcare. The case study methodology included collecting contextual data related to each case from four data sources, including contextual document sources, diary entries that detailed the creative contributions (idea-sharing and action), follow-up questions via email and participant-observer sources.

Reflexive Thematic (individual and cross-case) Analysis [3] enabled findings to be grouped into four themes. The themes are summarised as follows:

1. *Social position*: An individual's social position and related *social power* influences their social behaviour, including personal beliefs about what is possible, sensitivity and the courage to act and bring change.
2. *Workplace politics*: The local micro-political climate (group culture) and wider policy influences an individual's confidence to bring ideas and change.
3. *Social connections*: Social relationships and connections at work matter for bringing and shaping new ideas. A social group that is open to new ideas enables improvement and innovation.
4. *Education*: Education about local social and cultural (socio-cultural) influences on group behaviour and strategies to support individual wellbeing enables idea-sharing and action.

The study concludes by outlining the highly contextual nature of socio-cultural factors that shape idea-sharing and change in healthcare and supports two practice recommendations surrounding education to improve understanding about influential sociocultural factors and ways to create opportunities for idea-sharing and action.

In the face of increasing workloads, unpredictable and evolving healthcare environments, and growing demands to address emerging health service needs, innovation, agility and responsiveness are essential. In this context, individual idea-sharing and the resulting collective action can be highly beneficial [4, 5]. To meet these complex and dynamic challenges, healthcare professionals need strong cognitive skills in creativity, idea generation and collaborative thinking as part of their everyday practice [5].

My research supports that significant workplace culture change is needed in healthcare settings to improve quality of care, reduce medical errors, enhance patient outcomes and foster a healthier work environment for healthcare workers. Numerous aspects of social and culture-based factors that influence workplace behaviour and patient safety and care are covered in the following chapters. These include topics such as individual position, social and practice-related operational norms and normative roles, hierarchy, idea-sharing and innovation, facilitating a learning culture, improving wellbeing, and the politics and micro-politics of healthcare. These issues manifest through a number of behaviours and practices in healthcare, all of which contribute towards building the local workplace culture. For example, workplace gossip, bullying, unprofessional behaviour, tensions and power issues in the workplace all shape the norms and group behaviour.

My research supports that each person has the power to shape the sociocultural dynamics of their workplace, whether through policy decisions or everyday behaviours. By reflecting on how we use our roles and influence, we can identify opportunities to foster positive change. This book draws upon my research and explores those aspects and invites individuals to engage in reflective tasks and take meaningful action throughout.

References

1. Philp-Von Woyna L. A multi-case study to understand the ways in which sociocultural factors influence everyday creative contributions in healthcare and higher education by student midwives. Doctoral thesis. Staffordshire: Staffordshire University; 2025. Available from: https://eprints.staffs.ac.uk/8884/.
2. Yin RK. Case study research and applications: design and methods. 6th ed. Thousand Oaks: Sage; 2018.
3. Braun V, Clarke V. Thematic analysis: a practical guide. London: SAGE; 2021.
4. Denhardt RB, Denhardt JV, Aristigueta MP, Rawlings KC. Managing human behavior in public and nonprofit organizations. CQ Press; 2018. ISBN: 978-1506382661.
5. Cheraghi MA, Pashaeypoor S, Dehkordi LM, Khoshkest S. Creativity in nursing care: a concept analysis. Florence Nightingale J Nurs. 2021;29(3):389–96. https://doi.org/10.5152/FNJN.2021.21027. PMID: 35110178; PMCID: PMC8939908.

Understanding You, Your Fears and Abilities as a Healthcare Worker

Introduction

This chapter is about you, as an individual, who can make a difference to your own workplace culture and wider healthcare workplace culture. You will reflect on experiences and perceptions, including how you think about work, behave at work and the day-to-day events and practices you observe and participate in. You will gain understanding about how your historical life experiences shape your sense of self, self-awareness, sensitivity (towards self and others), fears and courage and how your perceptions of self are inseparable from how you experience and participate in workplace culture. Problematic workplace behaviours are widely reported [1, 2, 3] and examples of individual problematic behaviour are discussed, including cases of workplace gossip, intimidation, bullying and rudeness. Specific focus is given to how you might encounter and experience these negative behaviours, how people typically react and respond and how you can change and influence the response, to better address problem workplace behaviours. Everyone, regardless of their role has an important part to play in how people behave and work together. Reflective tasks help you to explore specific aspects of your own workplace culture, its unique features and what is good or difficult about where you work. Strategies and techniques are introduced that help you to navigate different social and team challenges in the workplace.

A Positive Workplace Culture Can Be Cultivated

Plato claimed that whatever is honoured in a group culture will be nourished and cultivated there [4]. This means that the behaviours which are rewarded or valued in a workplace are the behaviours that are encouraged by the group. These behaviours will grow, whilst those that are not valued or honoured will diminish. With this in mind, workplace culture might be better described as 'workplace cultivation'. Every

L. Philp-von Woyna, *Unravelling Workplace Culture in Healthcare*, https://doi.org/10.1007/978-3-032-11771-7_1

workplace collectively cultivates certain behaviours and practices that become acceptable within the group. Individuals (as part of a working group) play an *active* role in approving, praising and valuing certain behaviours/actions whilst disapproving other behaviours/actions. Through individual action or inaction, different types of social behaviour can be fostered, encouraged or shut down (stopped) by individuals.

When Plato stated that what is honoured in a culture will be cultivated there he was also suggesting that the behaviours we approve of, praise, value and encourage are the behaviours that will also be passed down to the *next generation of our group*. This means the behaviours we encourage, foster, value and approve of in the workplace will shape our workplace culture in both the present and the future. In this way, the history of the workplace and our individual historical group experiences become important to examine, when understanding current group cultures.

Historical Materialism vs. Individual Agency as Influencing Workplace Behaviour and Culture

Our historical experiences of group culture influence how we will participate in the group culture in the future. For example, if opinions and ideas have been unheard previously because a group culture does not value or encourage idea-sharing, we may be less likely to share our thoughts in the future.

Some theorists and researchers claim that group culture is mostly influenced power, including social powers, historical legacies and economics. This viewpoint suggests power shapes how we think and behave in the working culture of a group. In literature, it is known as historical materialism [5]. The theory receives criticism for being deterministic (power determines how we think and act) and oversimplistic. Whilst *power* plays a role in shaping how we think and act, in the local group culture, this theory assumes that power does not reside in an individual agency. Aspects of power (outside the local group) and individual power (agency) are both explored in this book as influential in workplace behaviour.

Workplace behaviours can be positive or problematic, but our individual participation (agency) matters. Individual participation in social behaviours, like gossip and bullying, influences how those behaviours are accepted, supported or shut down, in the present and future. It means how we act influences our workplace and professional group whilst we are part of the group and also after we leave. Gossiping and bullying are two social behaviours which are explored in this chapter in order to understand how our own and others social behaviour can influence workplace culture in positive or negative ways.

People Will Gossip

Gossip is an expected social behaviour in healthcare and can be both positive and negative [3]. Gossip is defined as verbal evaluative communication among individuals about another person who is usually not present [7]. That means the topic of gossip might be either positively affirming or negative. It is an everyday aspect of conversation because evaluating others (making judgements of people and how people act in situations) often forms the basis of communicating information to one another. Gossip accounts for approximately 65% of speaking time, so it is a behaviour that we can expect to be a part of everyday work [8]. Strategies that evaluate gossip in the workplace can help to identify whether the type of gossip we encounter is a behaviour we want to honour and cultivate or one which we do not approve of that is negatively contributing towards our workplace culture. Workplace gossip often reveals and exposes the culture of the group (the norms and ways in which people work together). This means gossip itself can be an interesting place to start when thinking and reflecting upon the strengths and problems within a specific workplace. Through listening to how people gossip, you may be able to gain insight into what problems do and do not exist and how some culture-based problems might be addressed.

Positive Workplace Gossip

Positive gossip supports communication of group expectations and helps to establish beneficial norms and practices. For example, a colleague may talk about another colleague in a positive way by saying,

> Did you see that Rebecca got the promotion as Lead Nurse? She definitely deserves that, she's always so organised and she is great at putting the patients at ease. She's also been making a real difference with her input into the patient forum to make sure patients have a say about the new service.

In this example, gossiping about Rebecca communicates support for her behaviours, and more widely it supports a culture that fosters these behaviours. It supports the behaviour, attitude and actions that might lead to a promotion because it is supported in conversation by the group. Rebecca prioritised and valued patients' needs and she ensured they had input into the development of services. If Rebecca is the type of person who gets a promotion in this team, the type of workplace culture is one where patients say how the service should develop, and their opinions are honoured.

Positive gossip in the workplace can be a powerful means of expressing what is valued and what behaviours should be cultivated. Leaders and managers are particularly influential in cultivating positive gossip and because of their position of power which often contributes towards decisions about who receives a promotion or what the criteria for promotion includes. The ways in which those in positions of power talk about others will communicate what behaviours they approve of. However, it is important to highlight how every individual's (including those who are not necessarily in positions of power) gossip in the workplace influences the behaviour and communication of others in the group. Collectively, the behaviour of many individuals aids in constructing a positive or negative workplace culture with its associated social behaviours. Box 1.1 provides some strategies you can adopt to bring about and cultivate positive gossip. These strategies can also be used to disrupt or respond to negative gossip.

> **Box 1.1 Strategies to Participate in Positive Workplace Gossip**
> 1. Initiate positive gossip
>
> Think about an individual that you value. Think about their positive behaviours, ways of working or traits that you like about them.
> Plan to share your positive thoughts about this colleague with another colleague/s.
>
> 2. Show your support for positive gossip
>
> Respond to positive gossip by extending the positive observation/discussion. This cultivates solidarity and support for positive behaviours. Respond to negative gossip with positive gossip.
>
> 3. Cultivate positive gossip
>
> Think about informing an individual when you have positively gossiped/talked about them or heard someone doing it and why they were a positive point of conversation.
> Plan to take a positive gossip topic that another person has initiated and cultivate it by sharing it with other people.

Negative Workplace Gossip

The purpose and root of motivation in gossip is often to achieve a sense of social solidarity, a sense of belonging for individuals, and to experience a sense of bonding with colleagues through informal interaction, regardless of whether it is positive or negative. However, negative types of gossip are a warning sign of organisational dysfunction and failure [9]. Negative gossip often reflects low levels of trust between colleagues, which may be linked to group culture problems of social disconnection between workers and their workplace managers/leaders as well as a lack of leadership from them [10]. When leaders and managers provide the team with insufficient guidance surrounding roles, responsibilities and expectations of work, there is increased ambiguity and negative gossip can surface [11]. Individuals might choose to negatively gossip as a means of gaining social support about the uncertainty of their responsibilities and poor leadership [11]. In healthcare, whilst role and responsibilities are sometimes clearly understood, negative gossip can also surface from simply not having the capacity to fully fulfil all responsibilities [6]. Negative gossip is associated with exhaustion, high workload, patient safety concerns and burnout [6].

Gossip can uncover areas of risk and concern from colleagues that have not been raised formally [12]. Therefore, gaining understanding about what negative gossip happens in your workplace can enable individuals to better understand problems and strengths among groups and the local culture. Box 1.2 challenges you to reflect on occasions you have encountered negative gossip in the workplace and to think about how it may be associated with your own workplace culture-based strengths or challenges.

Box 1.2 Reflect on Negative Workplace Gossip

1. Think of a recent incident of negative workplace gossip that you have encountered and begin by writing down answers to the following questions.
   (a) Who did the gossip concern? Was it a person in a more senior position or more junior position?
   (b) What was the topic of gossip? Did it mostly relate to communication, work-related tasks or was it personal?
   (c) What do you think the person sharing the gossip was trying to achieve? Did they share to gain a sense of support about an issue, to work through feelings/process change or to build their own sense of power?
   (d) Match your reflective responses to the table below to aid evaluation and understanding about what the negative gossip in your workplace could indicate.

Reflective point	What it could indicate	Possible solutions
It was about a more **senior person**	This can indicate that communication channels between seniors and juniors need to be improved and that a power differential (hierarchy) might be problematic in the specific workplace culture It may also indicate leadership/management performance issues	Strategies that disrupt power differences between senior and junior staff Strategies that build the strength of social relationships Improved leadership support and/or training
It was about a more **junior person**	This could indicate that the junior member of staff has limited clarity/has some ambiguity about what is expected of them, and communication needs to be improved about what is expected It may indicate individual performance issues. It is important to consider when gossip involves a more junior member of staff whether the gossip is actually better described as bullying	Improved communication and clarity of expectations and roles by managers/seniors Increased opportunities for junior staff to lead Clear recognition and management of bullying

Reflective point	What it could indicate	Possible solutions
The topic was about **communication** (what someone said/didn't say or communicate related to work tasks)	This suggests communication and possibly hierarchical problems in the workplace culture. It may reflect low levels of trust and social disconnection among colleagues	Strategies that build trust, connection and peer relationships Strategies to improve effective communication
The topic was focussed on **suboptimal work-related tasks**	This can indicate performance issues and/or a lack of clear communication about role expectations. It can also reflect an unsupportive team, low levels of trust between colleagues, bullying, or indicate there is an unsustainable workload or work-related burnout	Strategies to build team relationships and trust Strategies to improve communication Clear role and responsibility expectations Redistribution of workload/working planning/ resourcing Clear recognition and management of bullying
The topic of negative gossip was **personally negative**/negative about a person's character/ appearance and not work-related	This is bullying	Clear recognition and effective management of workplace bullying
The gossip was shared **to achieve a sense of belonging/support**	This reflects low levels of trust and cohesion in the workplace and anxiety about feeling support and sense of belonging	Strategies that build trust and sense of belonging Strategies that build relationships between peers
The gossip related to **organisational change processing**	This suggests leadership communication issues and culture-based hierarchical issues It suggests more needs to be done to support the process of change and to involve more colleagues in change decisions and process	Strategies aimed at involving people in decision-making and change Improved communication about change Compassionate leadership throughout the change process

Reflective point	What it could indicate	Possible solutions
The gossip enhanced a person's **sense of power** (this can sometimes be difficult to decipher, but a good question to reflect upon is, 'how do you believe the person wants you to view them?')	This can indicate both poor leadership, dominant leadership, culture-based hierarchical issues and/or bullying	Strategies to disrupt and challenge power-based issues Clear recognition and effective management of workplace bullying

1. What could the incident of negative gossip indicate about the culture-based challenges in your workplace?
2. What are the possible ways to address these challenges?

Negative workplace gossip happens when there are organisational culture-based problems that promote individuals to come together in solidarity through evaluative communication (gossip) about their own circumstance, problems with the organisation priorities and about others, particularly leaders or managers. Leaders and managers are often held accountable for what is honoured and cultivated among a group, and they are often responsible for managing workloads, staffing, bringing change and strengthening norms and rules in organisations. A stronger leader cultivates more positive behaviours and creates stability during periods of change by setting clear role boundaries, clear expected behaviours, and advocating for change needed to higher organisations or higher managers and through a variety of ways, building stronger social connections and trust between colleagues.

Change itself is more likely to result in gossip, both negative and positive, because individuals gossip when they navigate and adjust to new norms or expectations as a means of making sense of the new organisation and norms [13]. This is an important consideration in healthcare because organisations are constantly changing as a result of technological advancements, ageing populations, changing disease patterns, new discoveries for the treatment of diseases and political reforms and policy initiatives [14]. In addition, there is often a high turnover of staff in healthcare compared to other organisations and industries, as shift work patterns alter day-to-day, and there is a higher turnover of managers and leaders due to policy and organisation changes. Changes can be challenging for individual healthcare workers because it contradicts a basic need for a stable environment [14]. Organisations and individuals can take steps to create a sense of stability in times of change. This can be as simple as reviewing working schedules and teams in attempt to increase stability and improve social connections among staff.

The degree of stability for healthcare staff at work can vary, even within the same ward or setting. For example, I have observed senior staff responsible for organising shift patterns for a whole team prioritising their need for stability and predictability by placing themselves and those (socially) close to them on preferred shifts together. This is problematic because it creates a group of individuals with a more stable and supportive workplace whilst others experience less stability, more change and less support. These types of social organisation differences may create a type of social 'in-group' and 'out-group', commonly referred to as a social clique that promotes negative types of gossip that are often driven by power and/or to achieve a sense of belonging.

Formation of a social clique stems from a desire to avoid rejection through aligning oneself with others who you see as similar. When social cliques form, members of both the 'in-group' and 'out-group' may negatively gossip about the opposite group, and it can facilitate bullying. Differences in group stability and social cliques may promote negative gossip as part of socially processing differences and this strengthens group differences and segregation impacting teamwork and safety. Negative gossip offers individuals a type of informal social support, but it also often reflects a maladaptive way for individuals to navigate and control uncertain and sometimes ambiguous demands of the workplace. Unfortunately, negative gossip in certain social circumstances where power differences or in-group/out-groups are present can easily tip into what can better be defined as workplace bullying [15].

Bullying and Unprofessional Behaviour

In 2023, a report examined 87 accounts of bullying in maternity settings as described by 37 newly qualified midwives and 50 student midwives [16]. One midwife's testimony is provided in Box 1.3. Bullying and unprofessional behaviour were recognised, but the midwife felt unable to challenge the behaviour stating that she did not feel *'able to stand up'*. The same midwife went on to describe what happens if you do stand up to bullying and unprofessional behaviour explaining that promotion opportunities would stop, fear and anxiety rises, and you can become another victim of the bullying group.

Box 1.3 Testimony of Midwife

I've witnessed bullying and unprofessional behaviour [in my employing healthcare organisation] not always directly to myself… but [I have] *not felt able to stand up for them*. This is one of my many regrets. I've began to realise that maybe the women [receiving maternity care] were bullied as well, were they made to feel guilty for their choices because it didn't suit that midwife, or did they experience this unprofessional behaviour between staff or between staff and students? How is that ok?'…You *couldn't go to anyone* because the management was part of the problem, or were deluded by the senior bullies who knew exactly [how] to get around them… They [the perpetrators] *would openly moan* if you pressed the emergency bell, and if things resolved, [they would] *accuse you of being a terrible midwife* who was no good. [They] would then tell everyone at the desk and *if they didn't agree they would be branded a s**t midwife too.* [16]

In Box 1.3, *fear* played a part in the midwife feeling unable to stand up and challenge the bullying and unprofessional behaviour. Fear can often be related to how we view ourselves as professionals, our beliefs about our own abilities and our desire to belong within the professional group [17]. In situations where bullying occurs, the social climate plays a role in enabling and giving permission for the bullying behaviours to take place, but our personal fears and difficulties (that are intertwined with our desire to belong in the professional group) also make us vulnerable to accept the poor behaviours of others [17]. For example, a desire to be socially and professionally accepted as a student health professional shapes and influences healthcare students social behaviour and actions [17]. Therefore, social and professional acceptance of behaviours among a group and the fear that individuals experience are key aspects to address in the breaking down of problematic group behaviours like bullying.

Bullying is a social behaviour that depends upon the self-belief of power over another. The greater the perception of power the easier it is for an individual to become a perpetrator. Most often perpetrators *perceive* greater power over another because of their position (they are a more senior member of staff), they are more socially connected (their social power in the specific context is greater than the victim), they perceive lower self-esteem or confidence in the victim (which could be for a variety of reasons) or they perceive the victim as socially marginalised in some way (the victim is socially different to them). It can be beneficial to understand how bullies operate because the *perception of power* forms the basis of their behaviour, and so the most useful strategies will disrupt their perception of power or completely remove the power or confidence for them to act in those ways.

Bullies often make their victims aware of their perceived power and individuals often feel intimidation and fear as a result. The midwife's testimony in Box 1.3 highlights the fear of being branded 'a terrible midwife' which assumes that the bullies have the power to make that judgement (in reality they do not). The midwife also experienced fear of being humiliated at the desk full of colleagues who are coerced into agreeing or shunned into the same 's**t' midwife category. This is based on the bullies assumed power to influence other people. The midwife also experienced fear that raising concerns with management was pointless because management are 'part of the problem'. Again, this is enabled through a type of power, hierarchical power. Strategies that address the multiple levels of power-based assumptions are best to tackle these types of poor social behaviour.

The midwife who gave the testimony in Box 1.3 reacted in a way that most healthcare professionals do when they witness bullying and unprofessional behaviour. The most common reaction to witnessing bullying in a healthcare setting is for others to passively observe the behaviours (often with recognition and concern) [18]. This is referred to as the *bystander effect*. It means that for the most part, people do not want to be involved and feel unsure or fearful of challenging bullying and unprofessional behaviour. Bystander behaviours can be categorised based on whether they are *active* or *passive* and further categorised as *constructive* or *destructive* [19]. A bystander who acts in an *active constructive* way behaves in ways that actively defend the victim. A *passive constructive* bystander might approach an individual after an event to check they are OK and to offer emotional support. A *passive destructive* bystander will ignore behaviour or avoid getting involved, whilst an *active destructive* bystander will act in similar way to the perpetrator and join with them.

A problem reported in literature that occurs in healthcare settings relates to the process of *socialisation* (processing and accepting a normal group behaviour) in bullying and unprofessional social behaviour [18]. When bullying occurs in healthcare, the most common response from bystanders is passive, either in a constructive way (by privately showing social support and empathy for the target), or in a passive destructive way (by ignoring or avoiding the situation), but over time individuals may become desensitised and accept poor social behaviour as the normal group behaviour [18, 19]. This means that when new staff, students and trainee health professionals enter the healthcare workplace, they first witness and then become socialised (accustomed) to what social behaviours are acceptable or permitted in that workplace. This point may provide a crucial inroad for changing healthcare workplace culture because it suggests that experienced staff in a team may struggle to identify where the problems exist because they are socialised (accustomed) to the norms in a workplace. Experienced staff have knowledge about how things usually operate in the team and service, and it can be challenging for them to identify where problems exist so as to start addressing them. When new staff and students are supervised by senior, experienced staff in the profession, it can influence how new staff socialise into the profession (become like the existing culture). The education of supervisors in health requires investment to improve awareness of sociocultural factors influencing practice and care and to adequately prepare the workforce to creatively address challenges in healthcare.

Education to Increase Individual Agency

In the UK, reports and literature indicate there is an underinvestment in the preparation of healthcare educators and supervisors [20, 21]. There is inconsistency in clinical supervisor preparation and training, as well as issues with organisational support and culture [20]. Developing cultures that foster collaboration and continuous professional development may significantly impact the success of supervision and student learning, altering wider workplace culture [20]. Specific professional preparation for supervision and continuing professional development varies, but in the UK, there is currently no requirement for nursing and midwifery supervisors to understand and develop awareness of workplace culture and sociocultural factors influencing practice before supervising, mentoring and coaching students and new professionals in the workplace. In addition, there are no specific teaching, master's or doctoral level qualification requirements to become a nursing or midwifery teacher. In midwifery specifically, the state of midwifery education report suggests there is an underinvestment in formal training for educators with only around 10% of midwifery teachers at university holding a doctoral level qualification and declining numbers of midwifery teachers with master's level qualification, from 70% of teachers in 2018 to 40% in 2023 [21]. This matters for changing workplace culture because education plays an essential role in bringing about improvements and change where it is needed [17]. Improved education can aid in the formation of new ideas or approaches in healthcare, fostering curiosity [22]. Formal education provides opportunity to build skills in reasoning, critical thinking and problem-solving [22]. Less investment in formal education means fewer health professionals will develop influential skills in research, policy and practice at a senior, national level, and it may also reduce the quality of education for future health professionals including the ideas and changes they can bring [17]. My doctoral research found that idea-sharing can be facilitated and developed in education but that students were sensitive about what their peers and colleagues thought about their ideas [17]. In the study, they were less sensitive to what peers thought of their ideas and more sensitive about the acceptance and approval by senior healthcare colleagues. Students could develop confidence to become less concerned about what others thought of their ideas despite initially being eager to impress more senior healthcare workers [17]. Students wanted to be accepted by seniors in the profession, and this influenced whether they shared ideas or acted upon them supporting that the existing culture of a group and what is valued by experienced seniors in the group is highly influential in shaping how new members of the group (student health professionals or new staff members) act. New members learn from established members about what social behaviours are acceptable within the group and what behaviours are not [17]. Those who educate or supervise students were also found to influence student ideas and confidence in a similar way, illustrating that education can provide opportunities that build individual power and influence, to create change.

Building Confidence in Individual Agency

There are numerous ways to practice individual agency (to act) in ways that promote a positive workplace culture. When encountering challenging social behaviours, it is uncomfortable for everyone, and it impacts the overall workplace culture. Whether we are positioned as a teacher, a supervisor, a student, a bystander or in another position, our response can ignore (allow the continuation of), enable (actively support) or constrain (actively shut down) poor social behaviours. Here, three key evidence-based strategies are discussed as ways for individuals to actively address problematic social behaviour in the workplace. These strategies are intended to complement the formal management of unprofessional behaviour where that is warranted, but is not appropriate for serious incidents, such as assault, sexual harassment, stealing, discrimination and harassment. Instead, these strategies aim to build your confidence to take the lead (from your position) in addressing local social-based problems through local group action; an approach which, according to literature, is considered effective [23].

Three actions that individuals can take include the following:

1. Supporting others and shutting down problem behaviour—This involves giving support (as a bystander/witness) to your colleagues or sourcing further support for yourself or your colleagues (from social/local connections). It also includes taking consciously considered steps that shut down problem behaviour.
2. Escalation—This involves drawing on the formal reporting processes that exist, but also thinking about how the behaviour can influence the behaviour of others in the future. Escalation is the conscious process of thinking about where a cultivation of the problem behaviour might lead by thinking about issues more broadly, such as how it impacts a victim's autonomy, and the system-level factors that may be contributing towards enabling the behaviour.
3. Educate—This involves learning (as a team) about what is needed moving forwards, so that problematic behaviours are not repeated. It aims to improve the sharing of learning and an understanding of how everyday behaviours contribute towards the wider workplace culture.

Whether you are a leader, bystander or victim experiencing, witnessing or hearing about problematic workplace behaviour, you play a crucial role in each of the three areas that are discussed in more depth in the following sections.

Sourcing Local Support and Shutting Down Problem Social Behaviours

All health workers occupy a *position*. Position refers to both how an individual views their world and how they participate in their world, as well as their social position (social connections), historical and political experiences and personal values/beliefs [24]. Sociocultural theory suggests that a person's position influences their psychological processes (how they think), opportunities (what they see as possible) and affordances (the means) to act in different ways in response to their environment [25]. A person's position heavily influences whether they believe they can act to address a workplace problem and their decision to act in response to witnessed or experienced problems, such as intimidation and bullying [17]. The most powerful sources of influence on individual position (the way individuals think, what they believe they can achieve and the opportunities they see to contribute towards change, and act to address problems) are their social connections with peers and social acceptance by seniors in the workplace [17]. Social connection and acceptance encompasses both the type of relationship with colleagues at work, but also the number and type of connections outside the work environment [17].

Social connections can improve individual self-confidence and empower individuals to act and so make a difference in the workplace. The idea that social connections are important in creating and sustaining positive working environments is founded on a set of well-researched philosophical beliefs. This set of beliefs underpin theories of social constructivism that suggest we make sense of our world through social understanding and relationships which enables or restricts our thoughts, behaviours and actions. What we know and understand about the world is influenced by who we connect with (socially in private lives and working lives). Social theories suggest that what we believe we are able to do in response to encountering problems is influenced by who we know, what we understand and how we view our position in the world.

Evidence suggests that peer relationships, as well as relationships in and out of work, may help individuals to better navigate and address challenges in the workplace by providing more opportunities to build confidence to act [17, 26]. Conversely, evidence suggests that social isolation or less connection with others can lead to individual vulnerability, through losing trust and confidence in others and systems [26]. Social isolation can increase fatigue in others and increase uncertainty about own beliefs and identity [26]. In literature, this is discussed as epistemic vulnerability, a kind of vulnerability that comes about from isolating ourselves (reducing our epistemic position) whilst losing trust and confidence in others [17, 26]. Changing our epistemic position can happen through how many sources of information we have access to, how independent those sources are from each other, how reliable the sources are and how diverse the viewpoints of the sources are [26]. This means that when we have more social connections and more diverse social connection in and out of work, it can improve trust in others, teamworking, resilience, problem-solving and the types of contributions we believe we can make at work.

Based on social constructivism and sociocultural theories, sourcing social support to address issues of problematic social behaviour should come from multiple and diverse sources. This offers the best potential to build individual and organisational confidence and the resources needed to address social-based challenges, such as bullying and intimidation. It also aligns with wider literature that suggests bullying needs to be approached collectively by individuals, peers, leaders/managers, organisations, systems, policy and society [27]. A social-based problem requires a social-based solution. Understanding that bullying is enabled through multiple social means, and individual harm can be reduced through social means, can enable individuals who may be victims or bystanders (witnesses), to act in ways that contribute towards effectively shutting down poor social behaviours.

Box 1.4 outlines peer-to-peer strategies that can be adopted by victims or bystanders to challenge behaviours in the local context. More discussions about strategies like these and more social support for individuals can build confidence to enact them. Having these strategies in mind can also aid individuals in *cognitive rehearsal* (practising ways of taking control by rehearsing in your thoughts with what you might say to other people). However, it is important to keep in mind that addressing such behaviours should not fall entirely to individuals experiencing or witnessing these behaviours, but that it is essential for multiple levels of support across organisations, to disrupt or destroy the powers on which these behaviours rely.

Box 1.4 Peer-to-Peer Strategies for Challenging Problem Social Behaviour Locally

Repeat, Summarise and State the Impact

This is a simple and often effective way to challenge problematic social behaviour, such as rudeness, abruptness and intimidation, in a succinct and timely way. Further action can follow this strategy to escalate concerns, if needed

Sometimes perpetrators are not aware that their behaviour is intimidating. Simply repeating and/or summarising your understanding of what another person says/does is sometimes enough to help someone realise what they are saying is not acceptable [28]. At other times, it may provide the clarity you need about a problem to escalate your concerns about it

For example, in Box 1.3, the midwife described how colleagues would moan if someone pressed the emergency buzzer and would say the midwife was a bad midwife. In this circumstance, the midwife might say,

Repeat and summarise

'I heard you say a midwife who presses the emergency buzzer is a bad midwife'

Impact

'That makes me worried about pressing the emergency buzzer when I feel the outcome isn't always predictable and when I believe I need help'

Label the behaviour and call it out with compassion

This can include labelling the behaviour to both or either the victim or perpetrator

Labelling the behaviour can be helpful for the victim, who can sometimes struggle to identify the problem, and as with the point above, perpetrators are not always aware of how their behaviour comes across. Important principles to stick to when *calling it out with compassion* are,

 To consider power differences and consider finding a second messenger (colleague) who can help with the conversation if needed

 To label the behaviour without attacking the person or making broad statements like, 'that was wrong'

 To ensure timing is appropriate. Immediately addressing the issue may or may not be the best time, but as soon as possible after an incident can be most beneficial

 To aim to 'land information'. This means you are consciously aiming to bring attention the way that the behaviours were observed/experienced [28]

Document and do not gossip

Gossiping about incidents of rudeness, intimidation or bullying with the *in-group* (peers) may inadvertently contribute towards the perpetrators sense of power [15]. To avoid this, source your social support to make sense of situations and to give you the confidence to address situations from outside the group where the incident occurred [26]

Document incidents you witness or experience. You may or may not use this in formal reporting processes, but documenting what happened can help managers gain insight into problems and for taking appropriate action [12, 28]

Show support for the victim

The most common reaction for individuals observing rudeness, intimidation or bullying is to not do anything in the moment, because of fear or uncertainty about how to address it [18]

However, showing support to the victim by showing concern, comforting, labelling the behaviour, documenting, not gossiping with the *in-group* and/or taking the other actions above, you can contribute towards changing culture and workplace behaviour in effective ways that feel achievable

Escalation

Problematic workplace behaviours, such as bullying and intimidation can only be effectively challenged through numerous individuals working together to shut down the unwanted behaviour [27]. A crucial step in managing problematic behaviour in the workplace is through escalation of concerns and the subsequent management of those concerns. Escalation aids leaders and managers awareness of problems, improves relationships between colleagues, breaks down hierarchical barriers and supports appropriate solutions at all levels in the local context. Every individual should gain awareness of what to expect from leaders, managers and organisations to support a positive workplace culture. A clear understanding of your workplace culture, where problems exist and what could be the possible solutions can aid your contributions in building a positive working culture.

Healthcare organisations may struggle to sustain inclusive, people-centred cultures, but the actions of local people, taking local action in teams, departments and organisations, are the most effective way to build a positive culture [29]. Compassionate leadership is a key component in creating a positive, effective workforce, and leaders need the courage to move away from hierarchy towards more compassionate approaches [29]. With compassionate leadership, escalation is not intended to punish and discipline but to notice, understand, empathise, learn and find the best solutions. It creates a workplace culture that listens and takes *joint responsibility in addressing problems,* moving away from blame and punishment.

When a joint approach is adopted to address problem social behaviours in the workplace, it creates a safer team environment with higher levels of learning and innovation [29]. In contrast, workplace cultures that assign more blame to individuals create fear, lack compassion and restrict learning [30]. Compassion is defined as a sensitivity towards suffering in self and others with a commitment to alleviating and preventing it [31]. There are differing types; there is compassion that relates to self, and others that encompass the compassion we experience for others, from others and self-compassion [31].

Leaders and managers influence the workplace culture through how compassionate they are to themselves and others, but every individual can influence the workplace culture through practising compassionately. Individuals who are sensitive to receiving compassion from others and who witness compassion from leaders are more likely to act with compassion [17]. This matters because experiencing compassion from others and practising compassionately towards self and others is complexly related to depression, anxiety, stress and wellbeing [31]. Compassionate practice can be explained through four principles [32]. These are the following:

1. *Listening* with intent and fascination to individual colleagues successes, enjoyment, frustrations, challenges and harm [33].
2. *Understanding* the perspectives and experiences of people. This includes understanding that individuals experience an event/workplace in a different way.
3. *Empathising* with the thoughts and feelings of individuals.

4. *Acting* in ways that intelligently address or help the person. This is the most important task for leaders [34]. It includes the actions leaders take to help staff work more effectively, which may include acting in ways that resolve conflicts, or by providing needed resources and training [34].

In Box 1.3, the midwife who witnessed intimidation and bullying stated that,

> You couldn't go to anyone because the management was part of the problem, or were deluded by the senior bullies who knew exactly [how] to get around them… [They would] accuse you of being a terrible midwife who was no good. [They] would then tell everyone at the desk and if they didn't agree they would be branded a s**t midwife too. [17]

Compassionate leaders would be open and interested to listen to the perspectives of others, understanding, empathetic and prepared to act in ways that support people to work effectively. In this example, this would include understanding the harm caused and experienced, empathising and recognising the need for action in holding management to account. Holding leaders and managers accountable requires layers of support through organisations, their policies and regulatory bodies. Setting and supporting expectations surrounding leadership and management at all levels aids recognition of culture-based problems and can also inform local and organisational action. For health professionals working in the UK, compassionate leadership is both promoted and supported by regulatory bodies and organisations [28, 35].

In 2023, the UK's Nursing and Midwifery Council (NMC) placed greater emphasis on compassionate leadership, recognising its impact on staff wellbeing, benefits in supporting a learning culture and in improving patient outcomes. Sam Foster, the NMC Executive Director of Professional Practice stated,

> Compassionate leadership is critical to create practice environments that enable the delivery of safe, high-quality care for people. The impact of compassionate nursing and midwifery leadership ensures that leaders acting as behavioural role models create psychological safety, a learning culture and the ability for individuals to raise concerns ensuring that person-centred care is always the priority. [35]

Support from wider organisations and regulatory bodies means that individuals are encouraged to challenge behaviour that lacks compassion, helping to better understand problems collectively to address challenges at multiple levels. In Box 1.3, a compassionate midwife might raise her concerns in conversation with managers by drawing upon the expected principles of compassionate leadership. She could say,

> I understand that as a manager one of your most important tasks is making sure we have everything we need to provide the best care for women and their babies. I'm concerned that midwives are anxious about pressing the emergency buzzer because colleagues don't always react in a supportive way to the emergency buzzer being pressed. This is a safety issue that could affect how we work together and how quickly we can respond together in an emergency.

An expectation would be that the manager listens, understands, takes the concern seriously and *acts*. Leaders and managers can respond in compassionate ways that support a learning culture and improves teamworking. In this circumstance, leaders play an important role in establishing what behaviour will and will not be tolerated.

Education

Awareness and education about workplace culture, what can be expected in the workplace and what needs to be challenged, and how, is essential for every individual healthcare worker to understand. With widespread workplace culture-based problems reported in healthcare contributing towards poor patient outcomes and staff wellbeing problems, every individual can benefit from understanding more about how workplace cultures become established and can be changed. Workplace culture matters because individuals working in supportive teams with clear role expectations and good leadership experience dramatically lower levels of stress [36]. In addition, a positive workplace culture results in higher-quality patient care and higher levels of patient satisfaction [37]. In contrast, when the workplace is not supportive and leadership is poor, the decision-making ability of staff is affected, and poorer care is provided [38].

In the UK, education surrounding workplace culture as an undergraduate healthcare student is not compulsory. This is despite the UK's Nursing and Midwifery Regulatory body recently identifying culture-based problems existing within its own workforce [39]. They commissioned an independent review by Nazir Afzal OBE and Rise Associates to better understand workplace culture-based problems and stated they are committed to addressing workplace culture-based problems found [39]. They found unacceptable behaviours including discrimination, low trust, micromanagement and lack of accountability for delivering outcomes and concluded action in five key areas to establish culture change [39]. These areas include the following:

1. Leadership and management capability
2. Building trust, psychological safety and inclusion
3. Accountability
4. Individual and organisational learning
5. Multi-professional working

Whilst the strategy aims to tackle workplace culture issues within the NMC as an organisation, the principles of their culture-based problems and solutions are beneficial to consider in local healthcare and are covered in later chapters. Thinking about the ways in which we can *learn* from problem social behaviours and the action that can be taken to address them moving forwards can aid in changing workplace culture.

Summary

In this chapter, workplace culture has been discussed as influenced by you, as an individual, contributing towards building the working culture of your team. You have gained insight and understanding about how your interactions with your colleagues can support different aspects of positive and negative work culture. Social behaviours of gossip, intimidation and bullying have been key themes as have examples of social behaviours that you may encounter. Whilst gossip is an expected social behaviour in healthcare, it can be both positive and negative. It has been discussed as a type of verbal evaluative communication among individuals which is important for social processing of change and a way to gain social support. The topic of gossip might be either positively affirming or negative, but can provide insight into the culture-based strengths and challenges unique to each workplace and team. Strategies for participating in positive gossip and evaluating negative gossip to uncover workplace challenges were discussed. This included building skills in recognition of power differences, the need for social support, connection and sense of belonging at work, and situations when gossip is better defined as bullying.

Cultures that permit intimidation and bullying were discussed as possessing key features that can be challenged through a variety of means at the individual, leadership and organisational level. Education was discussed as essential in shaping understanding, learning and expectations of leaders. Strategies to build confidence through social connection, effective leadership action and learning were discussed as ways to empower action to address problem social behaviour and improve workplace culture.

The next chapter will explore the social roles and hierarchies that exist in healthcare and how this can alter perceptions, decisions and overall workplace culture.

References

1. Department of Health and Social Care. Final report of the Ockenden review: findings, conclusions and essential actions from the independent review of maternity services at the Shrewsbury and Telford Hospital NHS Trust [Internet]. London: GOV.UK; 2022. Available from: https://www.gov.uk/government/publications/final-report-of-the-ockenden-review
2. Nursing and Midwifery Council. NMC Register Leavers' Survey: summary 2024 [Internet]. London: NMC; 2024. Available from: https://www.nmc.org.uk
3. Department of Health and Social Care. Reading the signals: maternity and neonatal services in East Kent – the report of the independent investigation [Internet]. London: GOV.UK; 2022. Available from: https://www.gov.uk/government/publications/maternity-and-neonatal-services-in-east-kent-reading-the-signals-report
4. Smith T. Plato and education [Internet]. EBSCO; 2021. Available from: https://www.ebsco.com/research-starters/education/plato-and-education
5. Duffy F. Marx and historical materialism [Internet]. Ipswich (MA): EBSCO Information Services; 2021. Available from: https://www.ebsco.com
6. Georganta K, Panagopoulou E, Montgomery A. Talking behind their backs: negative gossip and burnout in hospitals. Burn Res. 2014; https://doi.org/10.1016/j.burn.2014.07.003.
7. Michelson G, van Iterson A, Waddington K. Gossip in organizations: contexts, consequences, and controversies. Group Org Manag. 2010;35(4):371–90. https://doi.org/10.1177/1059601109360389.
8. Dunbar RIM. Gossip in evolutionary perspective. Rev Gen Psychol. 2004;8(2):100–10. https://doi.org/10.1037/1089-2680.8.2.100.
9. Oliver C. Reflexive inquiry and the strange loop tool. Hum Syst. 2004;15(2):127–40. Available from: https://cmminstitute.org/wp-content/uploads/2020/12/Human-Systems-2004-Oliver.pdf
10. Ellwardt L, Wittek R, Wielers R. Talking about the boss: effects of generalized and interpersonal trust on workplace gossip. Group Org Manag. 2012;37(4):521–49. https://doi.org/10.1177/1059601112450607.

11. Hodson R. Group standards and the organization of work: the effort bargain reconsidered. Res Sociol Organ. 1993;11:55–80.

12. Noon M, Delbridge R. News from behind my hand: gossip in organizations. Organ Stud [Internet]. 1993;14(1):23–36. https://doi.org/10.1177/017084069301400103.

13. Houmanfar R, Johnson R. Organizational implications of gossip and rumor. J Organ Behav Manag. 2004;23(2–3):117–38. https://doi.org/10.1300/J075v23n02_07.

14. Nielsen MB, Finne LB, Parveen S, Einarsen SV. Assessing workplace bullying and its outcomes: the paradoxical role of perceived power imbalance between target and perpetrator. Front Psychol. 2022; https://doi.org/10.3389/fpsyg.2022.907204.

15. Kiefer T, Barclay LJ. Understanding the mediating role of toxic emotional experiences in the relationship between negative emotions and adverse outcomes. J Occup Organ Psychol [Internet]. 2012;85(4):600–25. https://doi.org/10.1111/j.2044-8325.2012.02059.x.

16. Burleigh A, Wylam J, Millar B, Gillen P, Webster J, McEwen K, et al. #Saynotobullyinginmidwifery: trigger warning – this report contains frank accounts of bullying behaviours and consequences [ebook]. Amanda Burleigh; 2023. Available from: https://www.amazon.co.uk/dp/1399969005

17. Philp-Von Woyna L. A multi-case study to understand the ways in which sociocultural factors influence everyday creative contributions in healthcare and higher education by student midwives [doctoral thesis]. Staffordshire: Staffordshire University; 2025. Available from: https://eprints.staffs.ac.uk/8884/

18. Jönsson S, Muhonen T. Factors influencing the behavior of bystanders to workplace bullying in healthcare – a qualitative descriptive interview study. Res Nurs Health. 2022;45:424–32. https://doi.org/10.1002/nur.22228.

19. Paull M, Omari M, Standen P. When is a bystander not a bystander? A typology of the roles of bystanders in workplace bullying. Asia Pac J Hum Resour. 2012;50(3):351–66.

20. Addis G, Loughrey N. Experiences and evaluation of the new standards for student supervision and assessment. Br J Nurs. 2025;34(1):36–40. https://doi.org/10.12968/bjon.2024.0334.

21. Royal College of Midwives. State of midwifery education 2023 [pdf]. London: RCM; 2023. Available from: https://www.rcm.org.uk/publications/state-of-midwifery-education-2023/

22. Li CP, He LP. Trait creativity among midwifery students: a cross-sectional study. Rev Assoc Med Bras (1992). 2023;69(4):e20221355. https://doi.org/10.1590/1806-9282.20221355. PMID: 37075447; PMCID: PMC10176656

23. Abou Hashish EA, Alsayed S, Alnajjar HA, Abu Bakar SA. The relationship between organizational justice and bullying behaviors among nurses: the role of nurse managers' caring behaviors [Internet]. BMC Nurs. 2024;23:503. https://doi.org/10.1186/s12912-024-02134-1.

24. Holmes AGD. Researcher positionality – a consideration of its influence and place in qualitative research – a new researcher guide. Int J Educ. 2020;8(4) https://doi.org/10.34293/education.v8i4.3232.

25. Glăveanu VP. A sociocultural theory of creativity: bridging the social, the material and the psychological. Rev Gen Psychol. 2020;24(4):335–54.

26. Kerwer M, Rosman T, Wedderhoff O, Chasiotis A. Disentangling the process of epistemic change: the role of epistemic volition. Br J Educ Psychol. 2021;91(1):1–26. https://doi.org/10.1111/bjep.12372.

27. Gaffney H, Ttofi MM, Farrington DP. What works in anti-bullying programs? Analysis of effective intervention components. J Sch Psychol. 2021;85:37–56. https://doi.org/10.1016/j.jsp.2020.12.002.

28. Royal College of Obstetricians and Gynaecologists. Improving workplace behaviours: workplace behaviour toolkit [Internet]. London: RCOG; 2021. Available from: https://www.rcog.org.uk/careers-and-training/workforce/improving-workplace-behaviours/workplace-behaviour-toolkit/

29. Bailey S, West M. What is compassionate leadership? [Internet]. The King's Fund; 2022. Available from: https://www.kingsfund.org.uk/publications/what-is-compassionate-leadership

30. Edmondson AC, Lei Z. Psychological safety: the history, renaissance, and future of an interpersonal construct. Annu Rev Organ Psych Organ Behav. 2014; https://doi.org/10.1146/annurev-orgpsych-031413-091305.
31. Gilbert P, Catarino F, Duarte C, et al. The development of compassionate engagement and action scales for self and others. J Compassionate Health Care. 2017;4:4. https://doi.org/10.1186/s40639-017-0033-3.
32. Atkins PWB, Parker SK. Understanding individual compassion in organizations: the role of appraisals and psychological flexibility. Acad Manag Rev. 2012; https://doi.org/10.5465/amr.2010.0490.
33. West MA. Compassionate leadership: sustaining wisdom, humanity and presence in health and social care. London: The Swirling Leaf Press; 2021.
34. McCauley CD, Fick-Cooper L. Direction, alignment, commitment: achieving better results through leadership. 2nd ed. Greensboro: Center for Creative Leadership; 2020.
35. Nursing and Midwifery Council. Supporting nursing and midwifery leaders to ensure the best possible care [Internet]. London: NMC; 2023. Available from: https://www.nmc.org.uk/news/news-and-updates/supporting-nursing-and-midwifery-leaders-to-ensure-the-best-possible-care
36. Lyubovnikova J, West MA, Dawson JF, Carter MR. 24-karat or fool's gold? Consequences of real team and co-acting group membership in healthcare organizations. Eur J Work Organ Psychol. 2014;24(6):929–50. https://doi.org/10.1080/1359432X.2014.992421.
37. West MA, Dawson JF. Employee engagement and NHS performance [Internet]. The King's Fund; 2012. Available from: https://www.kingsfund.org.uk/sites/default/files/employee-engagement-nhs-performance-west-dawson-leadership-review2012-paper.pdf
38. West THR, Daher P, Dawson JF, Lyubovnikova J, Buttigieg SC, West MA. The relationship between leader support, staff influence over decision making, work pressure and patient satisfaction: a cross-sectional analysis of NHS datasets in England. BMJ Open. 2022; https://doi.org/10.1136/bmjopen-2021-052778.
39. Nursing and Midwifery Council. Culture Transformation Plan 2025–2028 [pdf]. London: Nursing and Midwifery Council; 2025. Available from: https://www.nmc.org.uk/globalassets/sitedocuments/independent-reviews/2025/nmc-culture-transformation-plan-2025.pdf

2

The Problem with the Usual Way of Doing Things: Understanding Healthcare System Hierarchies, Normative Roles and How You Can Positively Challenge Them

Introduction

Healthcare functions like a system with a series of predictable processes and events that happen each day. This influences the workplace culture, including how people work together. For example, a typical ward day begins with handover (shift change) followed by a set schedule including times for medication administration, patient observations and other care-related tasks. Different staff groups work together, each understanding the usual schedule, process and what each person is responsible for. In some ways this makes working in healthcare predictable which can be beneficial for staff groups and patients. Good and well-established routines and schedules can make it easier to manage care and ensure medications are given on time and observations of patients are undertaken at regular intervals and can help with accountability by clearly identifying who is responsible for what task. However, whilst routines and processes have clear benefits for the management and organisation of care, some routines also lead to unintended consequences that sustain inequality and/or poor care. At times, established patterns of working can increase risk to individual patients indicating that there are times when healthcare needs to individualised and agile. By drawing on examples from public inquiries, media coverage and cases from my doctoral research, this chapter unpicks the roles individuals play in sustaining some problematic workplace norms, normative roles (who can and cannot act in their assigned role) and how these can be challenged to benefit staff and patients. By focussing on how the *usual way* of working in healthcare can advantage some staff and patient groups whilst equally, adversely affecting others, individuals gain insight into aspects of healthcare that need to be disrupted and/or challenged.

L. Philp-von Woyna, *Unravelling Workplace Culture in Healthcare*, https://doi.org/10.1007/978-3-032-11771-7_2

Examining Hierarchical Relationships and Normative Roles and Workplace Culture

A change in workplace culture is needed in healthcare to improve patient experience and outcomes, reduce errors, improve quality of care and foster a healthier working environment for staff [1]. Implementing culture-based change requires a comprehensive and systematic approach that includes examining the current ways of working and implements strategies that empower action from individual workers and change mindsets and behaviours of whole staff groups. The mindset and behaviour of individuals can be largely influenced by what they believe about their role (their perspectives about normative roles in healthcare) [2]. Individuals gain understanding about what is and is not their responsibility and what actions they are accountable for, in shaping their behaviours, mindset and decisions [2].

Healthcare practice involves patients and healthcare workers *acting* in different social and professional positions that hold differing levels of power and influence. From a human factors perspective, power differentials between professional roles, such as differences in perception about the weight of the opinion of a doctor compared to the opinion of a nurse or patient, is termed as *the authority gradient*. The term *authority gradient* was first defined in aviation when it was noted that pilots and copilots may not communicate effectively if there is a significant difference in their experience, perceived expertise or authority [3]. *Authority gradients* often mirror established hierarchical systems and roles. Understanding your position in relation to others, including what authority gradients or hierarchical systems exist surrounding your assigned role, is important because it can improve self-awareness and understanding about the decisions you make and how you think about problems, make decisions and act in practice. Established authority gradients and hierarchical social roles are sustained through the *culture* of a workplace. Culture can be defined as the traditional behaviour which has been developed and successively learned by each generation [4].

In healthcare, traditional behaviours linked to specific professional roles are successively learned by new generations of healthcare professionals who learn to imitate and sustain the behaviours of their predecessors in the field of expertise. This *socialisation* that builds professional identity and belonging collectively sustains hierarchical norms, resulting in differing *authority gradients* that influence the behaviour and thinking of individual healthcare workers. Several theories have examined how professionals assume their identity and develop as they become experienced through learning from others who already practice in the field of expertise. Seminal work by Lave and Wenger studied midwives to inform their theory about participation and learning in what they termed *communities of practice* [5]. This social theory remains popular in understanding how individuals learn in *communities* with common interests and identities. Individual behaviour reflects meaning that is given in *local communities of learning* by *experienced others* (experienced health professionals give value and meaning to how new health professionals behave) [5]. The experienced *community of practice* is what sustains and informs meaning, identity, and learning through observing and then participating in an established set of practices [5].

In healthcare, learning to accept the established *way of the community* means that new workers take on the assumptions about who makes what decision, in what role and position and where authority over decisions sits (who holds different levels of power). For example, normative healthcare culture gives different weight to individual health practitioners who are positioned in differing social-professional roles. This may translate to a doctor's opinion being perceived as holding more weight when compared to a nurse's opinion (as modelled by others experienced in the field) and the patient's opinion.

The true extent of culture-based healthcare hierarchical norms can be seen when individuals *shift* social roles within an established culture and ways of practicing. A recent news report detailed the case of Professor Patel. Professor Patel was a Consultant Haematologist who found himself in the unfortunate position of becoming a patient requiring care in his area of clinical expertise. In response to understanding the extent of his own illness, Professor Patel advised doctors and nurses caring for him that he required urgent treatment with immunosuppressants and he emphasised that time was of the essence [6]. The medical and nursing team caring for him decided on a different course of treatment, and Professor Patel's wife, a GP, reported that doctors expressed irritation at being given advice on treatment [6]. Feelings of irritation can sometimes surface when the usual (familiar) hierarchy or norms are challenged because there is an inbuilt conceptual gravity and preference for familiarity which can limit how we accept alternative views or ideas [7]. Sometimes, this limits how we can uncover solutions to problems because it can create perspectival blindness (we only see things from our familiar perspective). This can lead to losing the potential gains of considering other viewpoints and departing from the familiar, usual ways things are done. Usually, the doctor leading the care, not the patient, decides on the level of urgency. In Professor Patel's case, an inability to recognise and act on the expert's advice ended in tragedy when he died after not receiving prompt immunosuppressant treatment.

This case marks the poignant dangers of working in the *usual way*, limiting ability to work flexibly by providing individualised, responsive care. Box 2.1 provides an opportunity for you to reflect on Professor Patel's case further.

Box 2.1 Reflecting on Professor Patel's Case: Issues of Hierarchy and Power in Healthcare

Do you think Professor Patel's advice would have been received differently if he was the consultant reviewing a patient with the same condition on the ward?

What barriers do you think existed which prevented Professor Patel's opinion from being heard?

How do you think you could dismantle these barriers?

Professor Patel's case highlights the temporal and unstable nature of social-based and culturally constructed positions and roles in existing healthcare culture. It illustrates how perceptions about professional roles and position causes individuals to think differently about the weight held regarding the opinions of others. It illuminates how and why health professionals might respond to and make decisions differently, based on their perceptions of *position and role* in healthcare. If Professor Patel was the Lead Consultant for a patient in a similar circumstance, it is likely the team would have assigned more weight to his recommendations and acted upon them, but when his *social position* changed to being a patient, his power to influence care reduced. The social positions, patient and doctor are *socially constructed* roles in healthcare (built/constructed on social understanding).

Understanding constructed roles in healthcare aids insight into our own and other's positions and promotes openness that can alter how we work together (culture). Where an individual is positioned, at a particular point in time, can influence their receptiveness, courage or sensitivity to act in particular ways. Position in this regard not only refers to the issues discussed so far, our professional role, our position in a hierarchical system, but also it refers to how we view, perceive and understand our role, how we participate in our role, and the social, historical, political experiences in healthcare, along with our personal values and beliefs [8]. Position is a concept that is beneficial for individuals working in healthcare to understand because it can explain how and why the *usual way of working* is intertwined with our individual development as healthcare workers, our mindset and behaviour. The next section aims to challenge you to think about your own position in greater depth and to recognise and understand where you are positioned and the power you hold to influence the wider system and culture.

Recognising Tensions and Power in the Workplace

Professor Patel's case provided an example about how normative roles and hierarchical systems can influence an individual healthcare worker's perception, receptiveness and openness to take on board the opinions of others. To understand how and why health professionals respond the way they do in cases like Professor Patel's, healthcare system tensions can be further explored. A recent systematic review explored existing tensions in healthcare innovation efforts and identified 42 tensions across 29 studies [9]. Most tensions came about through dilemmas encountered during implementation of unfamiliar practice, such as conflicts between *standard practice* or standardisation and flexibility [9]. Tensions were also identified surrounding performance, old practices versus new approaches to care and clashes between understanding the identities of individuals and groups. Tensions are not inherently negative and may prompt change and innovation, but agile, reflexive approaches are essential to navigate workplace tensions [9].

Current established ways of working in healthcare include a number of ongoing workplace tensions which can challenge healthcare workers in providing safe and personalised care. This is not only evidenced through cases such as Professor Patel's but also through a myriad of recent healthcare investigations, inquiries, and media coverage that highlight hierarchical tensions and power issues in healthcare. In the field of midwifery, a recent UK inquiry examined the traumatic experiences of women during childbirth and summarised maternity care as a 'system where poor care is all-too-frequently *tolerated as normal*, and women are treated as an inconvenience' [10]. The report refers to what is 'tolerated as normal' in the established working culture and details numerous cases of traumatic childbirth that can be attributed to these norms. The report concludes with recommendations that outline a series of *system-level improvements* to address failures. Whilst system level changes are beneficial and are explored further in Chaps. 4, 5 and 6, system level approaches cannot fully address culture-based concerns because individual-level responses to culture-based problems are also required [2]. Throughout the report there are incidences of interpersonal communication and compassion failures. For example, one case describes a woman who felt her pregnant 'bump height had dropped 8 days before [her due date]'. She stated,

> My midwife had sent for a growth scan, but nobody contacted me to tell me the scan had been refused. I called up [the hospital] chasing it 44 times on one day but was just told there was a note saying 'scan refused, bring induction forwards', which nobody did. My midwife kept reassuring me it was her head in my pelvis, so I didn't know whether to be worried or not. (pg. 14)

The woman's baby subsequently died in labour and an investigation ruled that if the woman was given an ultrasound scan as recommended in the UK's National Institute for Health and Care Excellence guidelines [11], the death of her baby could have been prevented. Another case describes how a woman who was experiencing,

> horrendous urinary and faecal incontinence' was told by a consultant that there was nothing physically wrong with her, and that the symptoms were a result of her poor mental health. (pg. 14)

These two cases provide examples where the *usual way of doing and responding to the needs and opinions of others* in healthcare result in harm. This is not the result of one person's response, action or inaction, but reflects a plethora of tensions (from roles, resources, policies, hierarchies), working pressures and power struggles that may have contributed towards or restricted how an individual could have responded in each case discussed. It is beneficial to be able to recognise the tensions and practices reported, as workplace culture-based problems that can be influenced by individuals. Being *sensitive* towards the need for change at every level, individual and system, is essential for bringing culture-based change and ideas for solutions to problems [7]. Sensitivity varies between individual healthcare workers at the individual level; some are more sensitive in one way or towards a type of need and less sensitive towards recognising other needs. Every person working in healthcare may sometimes dismiss a problem, as not a problem at all, or accept it with an unquestioning attitude. Individuals may also lose sensitivity over time due to repeated exposure, leading to desensitisation of others' needs often with a narrative of self-reasoning. This can lead to existing healthcare culture problems becoming persistent, ingrained and sustained within healthcare. Box 2.2. prompts you to think about your own sensitivity as a means of prompting thought and providing insight into the problems that exist in your workplace culture.

> **Box 2.2 Reflect on Your Sensitivity Towards Workplace Culture-Based Issues**
> Everyday experiences in healthcare can prompt us to think and act differently in the future, creating culture-based change.
>
> 1. Think about a recent experience involving others that made you feel uncomfortable. It may be a practice you observed, or a decision made, or it could relate to a comment another person made.
>
>   Instead of simply viewing the experience as uncomfortable, think about how the experience represents your 'sensitivity' towards what change is needed.
>
> 2. What norms or assumptions contributed to how you feel?
> 3. Complete the following sentences:
>   This experience has improved my sensitivity towards a culture that needs…
>   At an individual level, I could address this by…

Sensitivity to Recognising Problems with the Usual Way of Working

A multi-case study examining student ideas for improvements in healthcare analysed the types of problems students were sensitive to [2]. This included recognising a problem, the process of seeing and thinking of an idea as a solution to the problem, idea generation and implementation [12, 13]. Understanding how individuals view problems and formulate (create) solutions is a prerequisite to every type of healthcare innovation [2]. It also aids in promoting a learning culture in healthcare. In the multi-case study, students who were more sensitive to identifying problems in healthcare were more likely to recognise broad culture-based problems, and shared ideas to disrupt norms. For example, one participant was motivated to share an idea because she recognised a power difference between women and their doctors when making decisions about birth choice. She shared a creative solution that could prompt and empower women to disrupt the power differentials by adopting a structured questioning tool which could be conveniently written onto a woman's water bottle. Existing literature suggests that tensions may prompt individuals to recognise (increase their sensitivity) that a problem needs a solution. Bringing-in ideas is often tension-laden [7, 14]; co-design tools (material tools to aid ideas like the water bottle) can disrupt norms and, in doing so, may transcend constraints in changing established healthcare culture [15].

Various types of prompts and tensions, such as experiences, observations and/or literature, can improve individual sensitivity to recognising problems in healthcare. For example, reports and media coverage, like Professor Patel's case [6], and a recent inquiry into childbirth-related trauma [10] can improve sensitivity to recognise similar problems and prompt thought about the ways the problems can be addressed. *Reactive creativity* is defined as the sharing of ideas that are prompted by experiences of tension (feeling uncomfortable) or trauma and offers a window into the underlying psychological conditions and emotions of an individual's relationship with the world and with the culture (norms) around them [16]. Some evidence suggests that persistent tension-laden experiences reduce sensitivity to similar problems or tensions moving forwards, which in turn reduces an individual's openness to new ideas [2]. This matters because it suggests that persistent exposure to tensions in everyday healthcare work can lead to acceptance of tensions as an expected *way of things* [2]. Student health professionals or new staff in a new setting may begin their careers *being sensitive to problematic practice*, but with more exposure they become less sensitive over time. Eventually, they become part of the practice they once viewed as problematic.

Reduced sensitivity, or perhaps acceptance of norms that are uncomfortable, can be a burden for healthcare workers, potentially contributing to symptoms of burnout and an increased turnover of staff [2]. Persistent tensions in the workplace are acknowledged as the most common reason (after retirement) that nurses and midwives leave the profession in the UK [17]. Maintaining, valuing and promoting sensitivity towards problems in current healthcare culture is an important step in making contributions towards cultural change at both individual and system levels. In contrast, desensitisation through repeated exposure to the *usual ways* of practicing might lead to an ambivalent acceptance and assimilation of those norms that sustain problem practices and inequalities [2].

The sensitivity required to recognise problems in healthcare is associated with human emotion, psychological processing and individual behaviour. Several recent studies focussed on emotional-psychological responses to the coronavirus pandemic, evidenced that emotion and purpose influence how individuals respond to problems, threats and concerns. Individuals were motivated to make a difference through civic duty, meaning they cared about society and people [18]. A further study found that individuals desired a purpose in societal action whilst using their affective (emotion-based) skills to support society [19]. Wider research supports that a combination of emotion and tension can motivate change and improvement through prompting individual creative action [2]. Healthcare improvements and innovation can begin when the *usual practices* and everyday events cause a tension or emotion to surface for individual healthcare workers. Therefore, reflecting on the aspects of healthcare that *feel uncomfortable or problematic* for healthcare workers is important to inform what change is needed. Individual experiences, beliefs about self and role position influence whether individuals decide to act on problems they feel uncomfortable about [2]. Many individuals who took part in my doctoral study demonstrated sensitivity in recognising problems, but only acted when they believed they held the power to make a difference [2]. For example, the idea of the water bottle (shared above) was intended to empower women who were receiving maternity care, to question, disrupt and challenge norms. The participant in my study explained that she did not feel as though women were receiving unbiased information and that their decisions were influenced by power differences and a hierarchical social relationship existing between the woman and the doctor. From this perspective, the participant demonstrated, firstly, a sensitivity in understanding the power, hierarchical and role-based relationships in healthcare, and secondly, she recognised the impact this was having on individuals and their care. Her emotive-psychological sensitivity prompted her to think of a way to challenge norms and in doing so she shared the idea of the water bottle, which could be used as a physical prompt to disrupt social power difference. The participant described the end goal of her idea as enabling women to 'question their care' and to help them to 'feel confident to ask further questions' to gain sufficient information about their doctors' choices. It is important to highlight that the participant was not only sensitive to the tensions, challenges and emotions of the problem she perceived, but she also possessed the belief in her own power to change the situation and the *courage* to think and act upon it through idea-sharing.

Courage Needed to Share Ideas and Bring Change

Courage is associated with individual and professional autonomy, increased creativity (more new ideas) and effective challenging of norms [7]. In contrast, conformity is associated with constrained creativity and supporting the *usual way of things* [7]. Evidence suggests that whether an individual feels able to act autonomously often depends on broader social and cultural factors, such as where an individual is positioned within distributed and dynamic social and cultural groups [20]. Historical experiences in particular (recent or not) are thought to alter a person's position (what they believe), their psychological processes (how they think about issues), their judgements and how decisions and actions they take are rationalised or justified to themselves [21]. Experiences of the world shape how we think and feel about problems. For example, media coverage that suggests changing healthcare culture is an impossible task, with toxic practices that remain unchanged despite numerous reports [22], can change what individuals believe about their ability to change workplace culture in healthcare. For some, this can prevent action and idea-sharing and lower morale and motivation, but for others it can increase their motivation for change. The direction in which an experience can lead (whether motivating or not) is largely dependent on the individual person and their other life experiences, beliefs, values and connections (their position/take on the world). This understanding suggests that experiences and exposures can alter how individuals think about problems and the solutions they believe are possible. What individuals believe is possible is intertwined with the power they believe they hold. A recent study examined the tensions in power relations, which included perceived levels of individual power and identity, and where and how an individual acts within a social context, so bringing ideas [14]. The study suggested that what an individual believes about their position within a system, and the power they believe their position holds, influences their *courage* to bring ideas to challenge the current *ways of working* [14]. This suggests that people only act to solve problems when they believe they can make a difference. It means that bringing cultural change (through action at the individual-level) requires more than sensitivity and recognition about what changes are needed, because courage is needed to progress from recognising a problem to actioning a solution. In addition to this, sometimes problems are recognised, but actions to resolve issues are difficult to identify. This is evident in a recent Nursing and Midwifery Council Leavers Survey that cites five core workplace culture related practices as the main reasons for nurses and midwives leaving the profession (excluding those retiring) [17]. The workplace culture-related factors were cited as burnout, lack of colleague support, concern about the quality of care for the public, workload and staffing [17]. Each factor in the report may be understood as representing a tension, but many are complex and multifaceted issues requiring collective action of many individuals working together to solve the problem. These issues can feel overwhelming for individuals, and so they may feel powerless to make a difference.

Culture-based challenges can be particularly strewn with tensions because tensions most often come about through dilemmas [9]. Dilemmas in healthcare in the UK represent a foundational and paradoxical tension between how the UK National Health Service (NHS) operates and British Cultural values. The notion of choice and its individualistic underpinnings is fundamentally inconsistent with collectivist NHS ethos, because whilst attempts are made to provide truly individualised care, it is not entirely possible whilst resources are limited and when fairness must be a consideration for all [23]. In pragmatic terms, this means that decision makers (about where a limited resource is needed most) are often doctors (not patients receiving care) and doctors determine and decide what defines a fair allocation of health resources within the constraints of the NHS system [23]. Attempts can be made to disrupt individualistic-collectivist tensions, but foundational problems remain and lead to questions about what choice in healthcare means when it is constrained by resources and the judgment of others. An example of this tension surfacing was found in my doctoral study. The idea of the water bottle (introduced above) was developed in response to the competing individualistic-collectivist tensions that gave rise to a creative idea. It aligns with empowering individualist British cultural norms that promote equality, choice, and liberty, but challenges collectivist norms within the NHS system where there are limited resources, and a system of hierarchy governs the fair distribution of those resources.

Conflicts and tensions such as those that come about through individualistic vs collective priorities influence the local culture. Individualistic cultures are more likely to promote creative expression than collectivistic [24], but individualistic ideals brought to a collectivist system cause tension, where efforts to enact individualist ideals through disrupting norms can be *squashed* by existing dominant cultural collectivist norms. Healthcare systems generally operate as collectivist meaning individual healthcare workers can find themselves in tension-laden situations where they wish to listen and act in the best interests of patients, but their ideals are *squashed* by what is possible within the collectivist system. This provides some explanation about how and why it can be difficult to disrupt norms through creative and innovative ideas within healthcare systems. If the system itself is underresourced and not able to provide the individual preferences for care (patient preference), it challenges healthcare workers who often want to provide the best care possible and preferred care for patients. Specific tensions in established healthcare systems (individualist UK culture vs collectivist culture within the UK NHS), physical constraints (what a patient prefers vs limited resources within the NHS) and social roles (patient vs doctor) bring a number of tensions that limit opportunities for change. Understanding these tensions and healthcare system norms, in this regard, is helpful to inform ideas. It highlights the importance of systems, healthcare staff at every level and patients having *ways-in* to challenge power with ideas and action.

Fostering Collective Ideas to Facilitate Culture-Based Change

Creative ideas to challenge power-based norms are needed as problems with power and hierarchy, and the fundamental organisation of healthcare continues to impact patient experiences and staff wellbeing. Theory suggests that idea-sharing and the generation of creative solutions to problems is influenced by four strands [25]. These strands include the *person* sharing the idea (their individual ways of thinking and personality traits), the *processes* that people are exposed to that encourage idea generation, the *products* that physically prompt idea-sharing and *press* (whether the environment is ready to receive new ideas). However, attempting to promote creative solutions to problems through one aspect of either *person, process, product* or *press* often means each is considered in isolation, but this limits how the strands interact [26]. Essentially, whether change and innovation begins with sharing ideas together depends on all these factors. The right environmental climate is needed to accept new ideas; people need cognitive skills to generate ideas, processes that encourage idea development and practical prompts and examples of ideas. Any aspect in isolation decontextualises how creative solutions can be generated and limits idea-sharing and change.

The ideas of individual healthcare workers matter for finding the best solutions to problems, particularly when problems are power-based and hierarchical, so efforts to promote idea-sharing from those who hold less power is important to foster, to effectively bring change. (The ideas that different healthcare workers bring are situated specific to their viewpoint from their own social position and how they experience the local culture.) This means ideas coming from different individuals reflect important connections between the person and context and highlights that ideas and the subsequent positive changes and innovations that come from ideas are largely dependent on what the social and cultural environment is like. Glăveanu's theory suggests that a person becomes an actor (one who takes action) by internalising the rules and norms within a group (the context) before being able to act creatively in that domain [26]. The psychological internalisation is a precursor to recognising where creative change can be made. Glăveanu draws attention to the multiple audiences (colleagues, peers and others who may accept or reject a creative idea) and the affordances (material potentials in the environment) that may lead to action and new artefacts (conceptual or physical creations) [26]. The theory supports the idea that an environment and conditions for the induction of ideas can be developed by thinking about how new ideas are accepted and what opportunities there are for all members of the team to contribute with new ideas. Glăveanu's later theory, the Perspective-Affordance theory, places further emphasis on the sociocultural influences of creativity supporting the interdependent nature between individual and social groups/society, psychology and enactment of creativity [27]. He suggests that sharing ideas for improvements relies on the bringing together of social, material and psychological factors and that a lack research exists focussing on individual-level outcomes and the interdependent social and cultural contexts [27]. Sociocultural approaches to promoting creative ideas pay particular attention to how creative action is made possible through living in a socially connected, material and cultural world [27]. It means that the people around you and the way people interact with each other create a climate that can support or challenge idea-sharing and change.

This contrasts with approaches where creative ideas for addressing problems comes from individuals, such as leaders. Individual views suggest that one person can produce an idea that solves a problem or makes an improvement, but in reality success is not possible because people in the team have to accept and act on the idea. In addition, whether the environment supports a new idea is also socially dependent (people act collectively to accept a change and bring about a change). Whilst one person could think of an initial idea for improvement or innovation, for it to be successful, the group must accept and act upon the idea. *Solutions are socially enacted.* This means social relationships, social connections and workplace culture (how people interact and work together) are *imperative to successfully solve any social-based problem* (including culture-based problems). The sharing of ideas among individuals, with understanding and an awareness of the sociocultural enablers and barriers that influence the success of ideas, is the beginning of culture-based innovation and change.

Sociocultural understanding is both lacking and beneficial to understand, because factors which affect ideas emerging from individuals are often influenced by their interaction in sociocultural contexts [28]. The perspectives of individuals interact and are deeply connected to others around them (socially) and also reflect their position in the world, what is physically possible from their position and what they believe is possible, as shaped by the cultural norms and expectations [27].

Perspectives are an important aspect to improve understanding about how creative action is possible, because a creative thought or action is thought to emerge from a perspective of uncertainty, disruption, dissonance or tension which prompts thought and emotion and the need for a creative solution [27, 29]. This means that when a tension or difficulty is encountered in the workplace, it may prompt a new idea, but exposure to different perspectives (from colleagues in different roles or positions) can further enable better solutions that are successful [7]. The best ideas for solutions to problems will consider a diverse number of perspectives from a range of colleagues, with conflicting views that may come from different people thinking of different ways to solve problems or improve healthcare can, paradoxically, help to develop new ideas. Research suggests that presenting people with conflicting perspectives can help them to think more creatively about the problem, and more creatively in general, offering more robust and comprehensive solutions [30]. In addition, surprising conceptual combinations presented to individuals increased their ability to think divergently [31]. The emergence of successful creative solutions to problems is thought to rely on some ability to adopt a different perspectival dialogue (to overcome our tendency for orthodoxy and instead move towards difference and divergence) [7]. In practice, this means there needs to be opportunities to hear the perspectives of many about culture-based issues and their ideas for solutions. Understanding the differing embodied positions can uncover what is possible (in material or action potentials) from differing positions in our workplace environment [27]. These potentials are made known to each other through opportunities to share and understand our own and others' positions and perspectives on issues [27].

Power and Hierarchy vs Humanistic Needs Influencing Ideas

How an individual perceives, thinks and acts can be influenced by their physical conditions (or material/resource available), social roles (or social status) and symbolic factors (social or political discourses) which affect their position in the world [32]. These conditions are partially under our control, but all can influence how a person behaves, including how they act in response to problems and the ideas for solutions they share [32]. Ideas for solutions to problems are always a *culturally mediated* [27], but regardless, expressing those ideas is important for individuals in their work and personal development. Abraham Maslow is a well-known humanist theorist in many academic fields, for his theory surrounding the *Hierarchy of Needs* that summarises what motivates people to behave the way they do in everyday life [33]. The hierarchy presents *levels* of needs that motivate individuals. At the lowest level, the theory suggests that individuals are motivated to meet their own physiological needs, such as food and water; followed by safety needs, belonging and esteem; and lastly self-actualisation. This is a diluted version of the theory because the original work placed particular emphasis on creativity (the bringing of new ideas/actions that represent oneself), as the ultimate human motivation (self-actualising act) [33, 34]. A self-actualised person is defined as one who possesses a mindset of openness and acceptance of self and others; is private, autonomous and *one who resists enculturation (to become like the culture)*; avoids problem-centring without solution; and has democratic characteristics [33, 34].

In my doctoral research, some creative ideas were shared, intended to disrupt cultural norms in healthcare, and were related to aspects of self-development, motivation and self-actualisation [2]. Openness to the ideas of others and acceptance of self and others was associated with more influential creative ideas [2]. The most influential creative examples proactively resisted enculturation (to become/assimilate the norms of the culture) and demonstrated positive, autonomously created *ways-in.* To create *ways-in,* participants acted with *creative courage, taking risks that ideas might not be supported by others,* with intention to disrupt norms. In sharing ideas, some individuals are more vulnerable to the opinions of others and wanted to socially test ideas before taking them forwards to share more widely [2]. One participant wrote,

> Prior to… [sharing more widely] I had discussed this [idea] with the people in my group. They said I made a good point, which increased my confidence to feed back to [the others]. [2]

The need to *socially test* ideas suggests increased sensitivity about what others might think of ideas and increased concern about rejection of their ideas [2]. Social approval or disapproval of ideas was found to be associated with either building or constraining courage and confidence in sharing ideas [2]. In addition, the expectations of others sometimes influenced idea development and sharing, because individuals want their ideas to appeal to others. This can lead to reinforcement of conformity to systems of hierarchy, power, practices and processes (even when these need to be challenged). This can unintentionally sustain ingrained views, norms and inequality and poor care [2]. This issue is explored further in Chaps. 3 and 5. Some participants had the confidence to challenge norms when they sourced social support through socially testing ideas. For example, one participant wrote,

> Having the discussion with the midwife first, made it easier as I knew she agreed with me, which gave me the confidence to suggest it. [2]

Seeking social approval or appeal suggests lower confidence and courage in bringing ideas but also highlights how the social and culture-based context can alter the acceptability of ideas. Some participants demonstrated high levels of confidence in creating *ways-in* and sharing ideas where they were viewed as *personally and professionally valuable to them.* These individuals placed high value on social input from others to develop their creative ideas, but were not as worried about how ideas might be viewed socially. One participant wrote,

> Being able to share these ideas is crucial. Not only can you ask questions [about how other people view things differently], but you can brainstorm ideas for solutions and use peers as a sounding board. This is especially important when it is difficult to engage [with others]… I often find that I am able to describe things in a different way. [2]

The social appeal and social acceptance of ideas influenced idea-sharing in differing ways for individuals in different positions. Openness to peer ideas produced the most feasible and influential ideas that resulted in action to improve healthcare [2]. This suggests that strategies and reflective activities that build confidence in one's own ideas, and sharing those ideas, can enrich collectively informed solutions to culture-based problems in healthcare. Box 2.3 prompts you to think about how you view and value the opinions of others and how this shapes your ideas and behaviour in healthcare.

> **Box 2.3 Reflecting on How the Opinions of Others Influences Your Ideas and Behaviour**
>
> Courage is associated with the confidence to share ideas, challenge norms or conform with norms. Think of a time when you have responded in a way *just to fit in* and to appeal to others or feel socially accepted. It may be that you did not find a joke funny, but you laughed along with others anyway, or that you did not agree with a statement or practice by someone else, but nevertheless you went along without challenging it.
>
> If you have been able to think of an example, then this is an example of when you have conformed to the social or culture-based norms despite these causing feelings of unease in you. It is important to recognise that when this happens and we try to *fit in,* at an individual level, there is a *compromise to self* which is connected to your own wellbeing and with the broader workplace culture. You join a narrative that is sociocultural-based that does not necessarily align with your own beliefs and values.
>
> 1. Think about how your example of 'conforming' at an individual level contributed towards the following:
>   (a) Sustaining norms
>   (b) How it makes you feel about your own opinions and aspirations
> 2. How could you respond differently to the same situation in the future?

Box 2.3 may have helped you to think about the ways in which you conform socially and culturally at work, enabling you to recognise how this alters your own thinking and feeling. This is beneficial in healthcare because individuals who practice in autonomous, thoughtful ways that are less conformist are less likely to contribute towards practices based on social acceptance and popularity (such as bullying). They are more likely to challenge workplace culture through making autonomous contributions that aid development of self and others. Opportunities for sharing individual-level ideas and thoughts in healthcare enables development of autonomous practice (among all individuals in any role in healthcare) that can challenge norms and break down problematic culture-based issues. In my doctoral studies, examples of how the *courage to challenge* develops through opportunities to socially test ideas confront health workers at every level to consciously consider their openness to others, especially those who hold less power, as well as how they can create opportunities to value the ideas of others. Individual healthcare workers can develop openness to receive ideas from both more and less experienced colleagues to support a learning culture, and to lead to improvements that are beneficial. In contrast, a lack of openness towards other's opinions and ideas, particularly from more junior staff members may lead to accepting problem culture-based norms. This acceptance and lack of openness in turn can contribute towards accepting (in part, at least) the inequalities and harms those problem norms cause. It also slows personal-professional development and healthcare innovation more broadly because individuals participate in sustaining problem culture-based behaviours. The next chapter specifically focusses on aspects of compromise and conformity and explores some of the difficulties in bringing your own ideas or opinions to complex situations that influence culture.

Summary

Sociocultural theory suggests that the hierarchical relationships and normative (social and professional) roles in healthcare can influence how change is possible through idea-sharing, improvements and innovation. The role of the individual in recognising culture-influenced practices contributes towards bringing ideas and change that benefits patients and staff. Reflective tasks and activities have prompted recognition of practices influenced by healthcare hierarchy, tensions, power differences and a desire to appeal to others in a social context. This chapter integrated insights from social, creative, humanistic, systems, linguistic and sociocultural theories, alongside research on human factors, recent healthcare inquiries and findings from my doctoral study. By the end of the chapter, readers should have identified effective entry points for influencing healthcare culture and developed targeted strategies for their own professional growth as health practitioners. The following chapter will build upon this foundation by deepening the understanding of self, shaped by the opportunities and dynamics present within healthcare environments.

References

1. The King's Fund. Improving NHS culture: organisational culture, workforce and leadership [Internet]. London: The King's Fund. Available from: https://www.kingsfund.org.uk/projects/leadership-and-workforce/improving-nhs-culture

2. Philp-Von Woyna L. A multi-case study to understand the ways in which sociocultural factors influence everyday creative contributions in healthcare and higher education by student midwives [doctoral thesis]. Staffordshire: Staffordshire University; 2025. Available from: https://eprints.staffs.ac.uk/8884/

3. Cosby KS, Croskerry P. Profiles in patient safety: authority gradients in medical error. Acad Emerg Med. 2004;11(12):1341–5.

4. Birukou A, Blanzieri E, Giorgini P, Giunchiglia F. A formal definition of culture. In: Models for intercultural collaboration and negotiation; 2009.

5. Lave J, Wenger E. Situated learning: legitimate peripheral participation. Cambridge: Cambridge University Press; 1991.

6. Tozer J. 'Brilliant' professor and father-of-two died aged just 43 after doctors botched treatment for a rare condition on which he was a national expert, his GP widow tells inquest [Internet]. 2024. Available from: https://www.dailymail.co.uk/news/article-13272953/Brilliant-professor-father-two-died-aged-just-43-doctors-botched-treatment-rare-condition-national-expert-GP-widow-tells-inquest.html

7. Runco M. Creativity: research, development, and practice. London: Elsevier Science; 2023.
8. Holmes AG. Researcher positionality – a consideration of its influence and place in qualitative research – a new researcher guide. Shanlax Int J Educ. 2020;8(4):1–10.
9. Haring M, Freigang F, Amelung V, Gersch M. What can healthcare systems learn from looking at tensions in innovation processes? A systematic literature review. BMC Health Serv Res [Internet]. 2022;22:1299. https://doi.org/10.1186/s12913-022-08626-7.
10. All-Party Parliamentary Group on Birth Trauma. Listen to mums: ending the postcode lottery on perinatal care [Internet]. London: UK Parliament; 2024. Available from: https://www.theo-clarke.org.uk/birth-trauma-inquiry
11. National Institute for Clinical Excellence. Inducing Labour: NICE guideline [NG207] [Internet]. London: NICE; 2021. Available from: https://www.nice.org.uk/guidance/ng207
12. Anderson N, Potočnik K, Zhou J. Innovation and creativity in organizations: a state-of-the-science review, prospective commentary, and guiding framework. J Manag. 2014;40(5):1297–333.
13. Craft A. Creativity in schools: tensions and dilemmas. London: Routledge; 2005.
14. Hyrkkö S, Kajamaa A. Distributed creativity and expansive learning in a teacher training school's change laboratory. In: Lemmetty S, Collin K, Glăveanu V, Forsman P, editors. Creativity and learning: contexts, processes and support. Palgrave Macmillan; 2021.
15. Wong C, Kumpulainen K, Kajamaa A. Collaborative creativity among education professionals in a co-design workshop: a multidimensional analysis. Think Skills Creat. 2021;42:100953.
16. May R. The courage to create. New York: Norton; 1994.
17. Nursing and Midwifery Council. NMC Register Leavers Survey [Internet]. London: NMC; 2023. Available from: https://www.nmc.org.uk/globalassets/sitedocuments/data-reports/may-2023/annual-data-report-leavers-survey-2023.pdf
18. Mohamad SM. Creative production of 'Covid-19 social distancing' narratives on social media. Tijdschr Econ Soc Geogr. 2020;111(3):347–59.
19. Karwowski M, Zielińska A, Jankowska D, Strutyńska E, Omelańczuk I, Lebuda I. Creative lockdown? A daily diary study of creative activity during pandemics. Front Psychol. 2021:12.
20. Rinne T, Daniel G, Fairweather J. The role of Hofstede's individualism in national-level creativity. Creat Res J. 2013;25(1):129–36.
21. Gelfand M. Rule makers, rule breakers: how tight and loose cultures wire our world. New York: Scribner; 2018.
22. Rimmer A. NHS culture change is difficult, not impossible – but essential, says health ombudsman. BMJ. 2023;383
23. Oliver A, Evans J. The paradox of promoting choice in a collectivist system. J Med Ethics. 2005;31:187.
24. Goncalo JA, Staw BM. Individualism-collectivism and group creativity. Organ Behav Hum Decis Process. 2006;100:96–100.
25. Runco MA, Kim D. The four Ps of creativity: person, product, process, and press. In: Reference module in neuroscience and biobehavioral psychology [Internet]. Amsterdam: Elsevier; 2018. https://doi.org/10.1016/B978-0-12-809324-5.06193-9.
26. Glăveanu VP. Rewriting the language of creativity: the five A's framework. Rev Gen Psychol. 2014;17(1):69–81. https://doi.org/10.1037/a0029528.
27. Glăveanu VP. A sociocultural theory of creativity: bridging the social, the material and the psychological. Rev Gen Psychol. 2020;24(4):335–54.
28. Lemmetty S, Collin K, Glăveanu VP, Forsman P, editors. Creativity and learning: contexts, processes and support. Palgrave Macmillan; 2021.
29. Beghetto RA. Creative learning: a fresh look. J Cogn Educ Psychol. 2016;25:6–23.
30. Gocłowska MA, Crisp RJ. On counter-stereotypes and creative cognition: when interventions for reducing prejudice can boost divergent thinking. Think Skills Creat. 2013;8:72–9.
31. Estes Z, Ward TB. The emergence of novel attributes in concept modification. Creat Res J. 2002;14(2):149–56.
32. Martin J. Positions, perspectives, and persons. Hum Dev. 2006;49(2):93–5.
33. Maslow A. Towards a psychology of being. 2nd ed. New York: Van Nostrand Reinhold; 1968.
34. Maslow A. The farther reaches of human nature. New York: Viking; 1971.

Are You Moving or Are You the Status Quo? Understanding How Movement and Diversity Supports a Positive Learning Culture in Healthcare

3

Introduction

This chapter invites readers to actively enhance engagement with diverse social and professional experiences and knowledge. It underscores the importance of fostering both individual and systemic learning cultures by cultivating curiosity and seeking opportunities to engage with culturally diverse movements. The concept of culture-based movement is explored through four key dimensions:

1. Opportunities to engage in theoretical movement (imagining and exploring how and where your own movement and actions and those of others might lead)
2. Opportunities to engage in empowering movement (using your position of power to make moves that empower others)
3. Opportunities to engage in social movement (deliberately making moves to better understand the roles of others and making moves that consider both your own and their perspective)
4. Opportunities to engage in physical movement (moving yourself to places and positions that are unfamiliar and maybe uncomfortable to understand more about alternative perspectives)

A key message in this chapter is that workplace culture problems are often local and solutions to workplace problems should come from many individuals with a diverse range of views. Drawing on global perspectives, sociocultural theory and organisational culture theory, the chapter illustrates how healthcare workplace culture is shaped by both local and broader influences. It emphasises how individual curiosity and diverse experiences can introduce fresh perspectives, foster innovation and drive meaningful change within healthcare systems. The chapter integrates cross-professional and interdisciplinary literature to highlight the value of varied experiences and viewpoints. Real-world examples from doctoral case studies and professional report analyses demonstrate how culture-based movement can lead to

© The Author(s), under exclusive license to Springer Nature Switzerland AG 2025

L. Philp-von Woyna, *Unravelling Workplace Culture in Healthcare*, https://doi.org/10.1007/978-3-032-11771-7_3

new opportunities, enriched dialogue and improvements at both personal-professional and systemic levels. Core themes of curiosity, openness, adaptability and resilience, at both individual and organisational levels, are central to the chapter's exploration.

A Stagnant Culture Versus a Learning Culture

A stagnant workplace culture is problematic for a number of reasons and can be characterised by a lack of growth, innovation and employee engagement, manifesting through high staff turnover, communication problems and low morale. In a stagnant workplace, individuals become more resistant to change and are inclined to practice according to the status quo ('stuck in their old ways') and motivation to innovate, share ideas and improve or adapt becomes limited. In contrast, a learning culture enables continuous improvement, autonomy and adaptability to change. In a learning culture, individuals are supported to gain new skills and qualifications and solve problems to improve care.

Adam Grant, a professor of organisational psychology, describes two types of workplace culture: performance cultures and learning cultures [1]. A healthcare setting with a performance culture will focus on the completion of day-to-day tasks and sticking to *best practice*, according to local policy and process, with less focus on innovation and the long-term professional growth of individuals. In contrast, a healthcare setting that focusses on building a learning culture encourages and enables individuals to achieve *better practice*. Where the dominant workplace culture is a learning culture, individuals are open to seeing and acting on areas of care that require improvement and engage in regularly sharing their insights whilst driving improvements. A learning culture supports opportunities for growth, sharing ideas and innovation, which may include enabling continuous improvement, commitment to staff development, research and innovative practices [2]. Despite evidence supporting that a learning culture at work can enable improvements in healthcare and staff development, culture often remains a barrier to improving patient care and outcomes.

Understanding Perspectives About Workplace Culture as an Individual and Socially Constructed Concept

To understand how a stagnant culture can be a barrier to healthcare innovation and establishing a more learning-focussed culture, two fundamental tensions in workplace culture can be examined [1]. These fundamental tensions in work culture relate to analysing the results vs. relationships and rules vs. risk. Individuals are encouraged to engage in conscious reflection on workplace expectations, with emphasis placed on outcomes, the value attributed to interpersonal relationships, adherence to organisational policies and the degree of autonomy and risk tolerance permitted. Perceptions of the workplace may vary significantly among individuals, shaped not only by their own social and professional identities but also by the attitudes and beliefs of influential others within their environment. People like to be socially accepted within their professional teams, especially by seniors, and at times, this can influence how they respond through their own behaviours and practices. Workers may seek to understand what the experienced people in the team value and then change their own behaviour and actions accordingly. In doing so, individuals are making attempts to *fit in* and to impress influential, experienced people within the team. During this process, they become socialised to (become like) existing culture. The idea that different professionals and workers become socialised into profession-specific value systems and established accepted norms in that profession, including acceptable autonomy and behaviour, can be explained by Social Learning Theory [3]. Social Learning Theory suggests that local communities influence how we think and act. Health professionals train and learn from *experienced others*, and this can explain why groups of professionals often have behaviours and traits in common. Social learning (learning from others in the profession) can create, sustain and inform individual and group meaning, identity and learning [3]. The process of 'becoming like' the existing working culture of a group/community builds individual professional identity and gives purpose and meaning to one's own work and endeavours [3]. When the professional culture is good, such as one which can be defined as a learning culture, the process of socialisation is beneficial because it strengthens the dominant cultural norms, but when the workplace culture or professional culture is poor, becoming like the existing culture can exacerbate problems and sustain poor practice.

Workplace culture can be different across both health professional groups and in different healthcare organisations and settings. Each team or area can have a different dominant culture type, and when new and emerging professionals join the team, they become like the established team working in the area, and consequently they can perpetuate social strengths and problems. The strongest behavioural features of the group are often perpetuated, unless the culture is disrupted in some way. One effective approach to transforming group workplace culture is to support individuals in exploring and experiencing diversity within team cultures. Research examining heterogeneity (differences) in healthcare workplace environments indicates that exposure to cultural diversity fosters more positive working relationships and enhances the quality of care [4]. Meaningful cultural change in healthcare requires a deep engagement with the diverse nature of the sector—both in its structural composition and in the ways professionals collaborate within it [4]. This includes recognising the varied approaches to teamwork, understanding the dynamics of interprofessional collaboration and developing greater insights into the roles and perspectives of others within the healthcare system. By intentionally and curiously seeking opportunities to learn about both one's own workplace culture and those that differ, individuals and teams can be empowered to work more effectively across diverse settings. There is much to be gained from engaging with colleagues in different roles and teams.

Exploring Your Own Beliefs About Workplace Culture

Exploring beliefs about your own workplace culture can help you to understand why team members behave and respond in the ways you witness on a day-to-day basis at work. This understanding can better equip you to challenge poor workplace culture and promote good practices. Literature suggests that to understand our own workplace culture and how this may differ from other workplace cultures, individuals can engage in reflective tasks that seek to examine and measure what is believed about the dominant working norms and attitudes in your team. A well-researched method of engaging with workplace culture reflection is through adopting a validated and standardised measure of organisational culture known as the Competing Values Framework (CVF) [5]. The CVF suggests there are always dominant culture-based practices in the workplace, and these can be understood by examining alignment with how flexible or stable organisations/teams are and whether they are more internally or externally focussed [5]. An organisational/team culture can either be more flexible and dynamic, or it can be more stable and demanding of compliance with hierarchies, rules and policies. In addition, it might be more focussed on internal values that emphasise care and commitment to individual wellbeing, or more focussed on external values such as measurable goals and competitive key performance indicators [5]. These dominant features of workplace culture can provide insight into the potential strengths and limitations of working within a specific team. Whilst dominant traits of the workplace might cover all four areas to some degree, there are often *more dominant* and *less dominant* features among teams and organisations.

Perceptions of workplace culture can vary significantly depending on the individual experiences and interpretations of who is asked. From a constructivist standpoint, these personal beliefs collectively shape and sustain the culture of a team or organisation. Consequently, a collective shift in individual perspectives has the potential to drive meaningful cultural change within the workplace. This means that personal beliefs about workplace culture, and the actions individuals take in response, actively contribute towards the dominant behaviours and norms within the organisation. For instance, if an individual prioritises performance metrics over staff wellbeing, they may expect colleagues to meet measurable standards, even when doing so compromises personal health. In a healthcare setting, this could manifest as staff feeling obligated to skip breaks during periods of understaffing. Whilst the expectation to maintain patient care persists, such practices undermine staff wellbeing and contribute to a problematic culture. This not only affects morale and patient safety but also perpetuates systemic issues like chronic understaffing. Individuals working as part of this team may uphold the practice by shutting down people who make complaints about insufficient breaks, which facilitates continuation of the practice. Alternatively, when staff wellbeing is recognised as essential to maintaining a safe and resilient workforce, and practices such as taking regular breaks are prioritised, a more supportive workplace culture can emerge. This approach helps workforce managers and planning teams better understand and respond to the resource needs of staff. It also fosters a culture that respects the collective wellbeing of employees, whilst reinforcing the importance of patient safety.

Understanding your own perceptions and experiences of workplace culture can inform how culture change might be achieved. Box 3.1 provides an opportunity for you to reflect on your personal beliefs about workplace culture. This reflection serves as a foundation for identifying potential barriers and enablers within your organisational environment.

Box 3.1 Reflect on Your Personal Perceptions and Beliefs About Workplace Culture

1. Consider the four organisational culture statements below. Which one or two best represent the culture of your current workplace?

   Statement 1: In a hierarchy-driven organisation, the workplace is highly formal and structured, with bureaucratic procedures guiding employee actions.

   Statement 2: In an organisation where adhocracy prevails, the environment is dynamic and entrepreneurial, and individuals are encouraged to take risks.

   Statement 3: In a clan-oriented culture, the workplace is characterised by warmth and care, with a strong emphasis on nurturing each employee's potential.

   Statement 4: In a market-driven culture, the focus is on competition and achievement, with measurable goals taking precedence [5].

   Reflecting on these statements can help you better understand your perceptions of workplace culture and identify areas for potential improvement. Statements 1 and 2 represent contrasting cultural orientations; if your workplace aligns more closely with Statement 1, introducing behaviours associated with Statement 2 may foster greater flexibility and innovation. Similarly, Statements 3 and 4 are interconnected; if your organisation reflects the characteristics of Statement 4, incorporating elements from Statement 3 may enhance collaboration and support.

2. What are the culture-based strengths and challenges in your team and what priorities do you consider essential for changing the workplace culture?

   Whilst this is a simplified framework for evaluating workplace culture, it offers a useful starting point for deeper reflection and strategic development.

Healthcare Is Uniquely Diverse

Research that sits outside the healthcare industry suggests that strong cultures often have very clear dominant characteristics, and there is often high agreement between core values, which can be advantageous in stable environments, but not in unpredictable or changing workplaces [6]. Healthcare is a dynamic and often unpredictable environment, where increasing access to diverse opportunities and skill sets can enhance organisational agility, teamwork, outcomes and overall experiences. In this context, it is essential for healthcare leaders and professionals to first reflect on their own beliefs about workplace culture and then to recognise the critical role that diversity in skills and across teams, services and specialities plays in effectively meeting patient needs. The concept of culture-based heterogeneity refers to the extent to which cultural norms and beliefs differ among individuals within the same broader group [7]. In healthcare, this overarching group comprises numerous subgroups of teams, professionals, departments and so on, each with distinct norms, practices, beliefs and areas of expertise. These subgroups are further composed of professionals with specialised skills and unique ways of working. Whilst this diversity can be a powerful asset, fostering innovation and adaptability, it can also present challenges that impact workplace culture. Understanding and harnessing the inherent complexity is key to building more inclusive, responsive and resilient healthcare systems. By completing Box 3.1, you will have gained some understanding about how you view your own workplace culture and what you understand its dominant traits and features to be. If your views agree with how everyone at your workplace views the culture, then collectively it introduces culture-based problems because each type of dominant culture has disadvantages, as well as advantages. For instance, if everyone views healthcare as an organisation that is hierarchical and believes the healthcare environment should be hierarchical, then the organisation will not be very adaptable or innovative [5]. When a hierarchical-type culture is too dominant, it may present problems where everyone agrees with and conforms to those in the highest positions of power. Box 3.2 provides an example of the serious consequences that might result from hierarchical dominant cultures.

Box 3.2 The Gosport War Memorial Hospital Review [8]

In 2018, a report was published that detailed the serious case review into failings at UK-based Gosport War Memorial Hospital. The case review found that the institutionalised (agreed and accepted) culture enabled a regular (normative) practice where the lives of patients were shortened through the prescribing and administering of opioid medications without medical justification. Reports detailed how 456 patients had their lives unnecessarily shortened because questions about the practice raised by nurses working on the unit were shut down and ignored. The established dominant culture at Gosport War Memorial Hospital was reported to have lasted over a decade and problematic practices were ultimately sustained by individuals joining, agreeing with and becoming like the established culture. Individuals accepted and actively supported *the way things are done*, resulting in concerns being ignored and unsafe practices remaining unchallenged. The dominant culture at Gosport War Memorial Hospital was hierarchical, meaning the workplace was very formalised and structured, with power clearly established and enacted.

Cultures with hierarchical dominant norms often dismiss people who wish to challenge the accepted norms. Dismissing concerns becomes easy because the power difference between members of the team is so great. In this report [8], nurses raised concerns about probable overdoses of opioids, but the lead doctor responded by saying that it was his normal practice. Whilst the nurse raising the concern knew that other similar units did not use diamorphine (opioid) as extensively, her concerns where ignored and dismissed because the culture allowed and even enabled it.

Understanding Your Dominant Workplace Culture

When social-based problems are encountered in healthcare, it can be helpful to think about what the dominant behaviours indicate and to imagine and explore where your own action (or inaction) and the action of others might lead. This is because an understanding of how social behaviours feed into culturally embedded practices can inform how those problems can be challenged through gaining an understanding of the factors that are sustaining them.

As illustrated in the scenario in Box 3.2, individuals may sometimes recognise problematic behaviours but feel compelled to suppress their concerns due to the prevailing acceptance of those behaviours by others. This dynamic can make it challenging to identify effective ways to question or shift the dominant workplace culture. In the example provided, the ward team operated within a hierarchical culture. One potential strategy for cultural change involves introducing elements of an opposing cultural model, such as adhocracy which encourages innovation, flexibility and risk-taking. Practically, this could involve envisioning alternative approaches to addressing the issue and taking deliberate actions that challenge unquestioned hierarchical norms, thereby fostering a more dynamic and responsive workplace environment. In part, the lack of diversity in culture contributed to patient deaths, with the dominant culture supporting and sustaining the *hierarchical-based power.* When groups culture reflects hierarchical dominant behaviours, there is a preference to have structured ways of working and clear boundaries about what should/can happen and what cannot [5].

Challenging dominant workplace cultures, such as hierarchical structures commonly found in healthcare, can be difficult, as illustrated in the serious case review example (Box 3.2). Equally, identifying how such cultures might be disrupted or diversified to address these challenges is complex. However, a key insight from my doctoral research indicates that problematic dominant cultures, particularly those lacking diversity and presenting persistent challenges, can be effectively questioned during the early stages of professional socialisation [2]. The study, which involved healthcare students, revealed that individuals often begin to form ideas about improving care during the critical period when they are learning to adapt to and align with the prevailing workplace culture [2]. During this time, participants expressed a strong desire for acceptance and belonging within the established professional group, and their actions, opinions and ideas were frequently shaped by what they believed experienced professionals expected or valued [2]. Many participants reported feelings of uncertainty and anxiety about how their ideas might be received, seeking reassurance and validation from more senior colleagues. This desire highlights how early *socialisation* can reinforce existing cultural issues. The findings suggest that this formative period presents a valuable opportunity to introduce alternative perspectives and promote cultural change from within [2].

Thinking Differently About Culture-Based Problems in Healthcare

There is often an inherent tendency to gravitate toward the familiar, which can lead to a desire to conform in the workplace and limit our openness to new or different perspectives [9]. This inclination can hinder problem-solving by creating perspectival blindness and a restricted view, shaped by our own familiar experiences. As a result, we may overlook valuable insights that come from considering alternative viewpoints or breaking away from established practices. Perspectival blindness can also cause individuals to undervalue what they could learn from others, assuming their own methods are already optimal. When we believe our current ways of working are sufficient, we may become less receptive to other ideas and more likely to reinforce our own thinking. However, openness to different perspectives is critical for meaningful cultural change. In my doctoral research, one participant recounted an instance where an idea she found useful was dismissed by her peers. She shared:

> I just felt they [other peers] would benefit from it as I found it so helpful, [but] two members of my learning set were not interested [2].

The example highlights what can happen when people have different opinions about what could work, and what they believe will not work, when attempting to find solutions. There is a perspectival tension (a difference between views about what could work to solve a problem) and a lack of openness by peers to accept or explore new ideas proposed. A reluctance to acknowledge the value and benefits of a different perspective can be viewed as failure to see the powerful discoveries that emerge from differences [2].

Sometimes, failing to fully consider alternative viewpoints or solutions can resemble a form of minimisation, which can be likened to overlooking and undervaluing the importance of different perspectives. However, the dissonance caused by contrasting viewpoints can actually stimulate innovation and lead to more effective problem-solving [10]. Similarly, other literature supports this view, suggesting that engaging with antinomy, the tension between seemingly incompatible perspectives, can help individuals confront challenges and grow in their ability to value and understand alternative ways of thinking [9]. In practical terms, this means that actively seeking out diverse perspectives within the workplace, and understanding how different individuals perceive potential solutions, is likely to result in more meaningful and sustainable change. Moreover, when people feel psychologically safe to express their views, it nurtures a positive learning culture, where contributions from all members are acknowledged and appreciated [11]. Amy Edmondson, a professor of leadership and management at Harvard Business School, emphasises that the workplace should be a psychologically safe environment where individuals can raise questions, share concerns, discuss mistakes and offer ideas without fear. Whilst psychological safety may still give rise to conflict because differing viewpoints often clash, such conflict is essential for prompting new ways forward. It creates space for honest dialogue, empowers employees to contribute and leads to stronger outcomes through the integration of diverse ideas [11]. In contrast, workplaces that discourage open expression risk developing a culture of fear and stagnation, where dominant narratives go unchallenged and innovation is stifled.

A useful perspective describes viewpoints as relational constructs that are shaped by who we are, our experiences, how we think, our social context and our work environment [12]. From this perspective, diversity in thought and background enhances openness and encourages better problem-solving [12]. When openness is lacking, teams may become less tolerant of differing views and more resistant to alternative approaches, whereas deliberately broadening the range of perspectives we engage can be important for addressing culture-specific challenges in healthcare.

Insights from safety-critical industries outside of healthcare can offer valuable lessons. For instance, in aviation, air traffic controllers play a vital role in ensuring safe and efficient aircraft movement, and they operate under highly optimised conditions. Their work schedules are designed to reduce fatigue and enhance focus, with mandatory 15-minute breaks every 90–120 minutes, shorter shift durations compared to healthcare and the support of an assistant to double-check decisions [13]. Adopting and adapting strategies from other high-risk sectors, like air traffic control, can deepen our understanding of risk management, safety and learning in healthcare. This cross-sector approach can ultimately lead to more effective and innovative solutions to the complex problems healthcare teams face.

Box 3.3 helps you to consider how differing perspectives can be beneficial in finding solutions to problems and in creating a psychologically safe workplace that supports solutions in an open, learning culture.

Box 3.3 Differing Perspectives Lead to Stronger Teams, Safer, More Effective Care and Better Solutions to Problems

In my doctoral research, which involved a multi-case study, I found several examples demonstrating how diverse perspectives and varied team relationships contributed to more effective problem-solving, enhanced patient safety and care and strengthened psychological safety and confidence among team members. The following two cases highlight how diverse working relationships and broadened viewpoints can support the development of effective solutions.

Case 1 illustrates how diverse relationships helped to grow ideas. A participant wrote about an idea that questioned a patient (safely) about her experience of domestic violence, whilst her partner was away at a hospital appointment. She stated that she,

> …was able to show the woman to the toilets…[and] because it was a multi stall toilet for females, I was able to take her and to 'fill up the basket for urine pots. This gave me the ability to ensure she was on her own and discuss things [2].

The participant *shared [the idea] across WhatsApp messages [with her supervisor]*, and it enabled her idea to be adopted among the wider team. The participant shared that her idea was adopted by others in 'other buildings and clinic locations' demonstrating the impact of her idea. In this case, diverse connections between clinic locations and staff facilitated the sharing and wider adoption of the idea. Through established diverse networks, her idea gained momentum and power and contributed towards transformational practice, beyond her own singular enactment in the specific circumstance.

Case 2 illustrates how diverse perspectives can develop and improve ideas for solutions. A participant experienced uncertainty about how to address a problem and utilise her diverse network of peers to find a better solution. She wrote,

> I…[firstly] created a mind map of issues... about how I could create something to turn [the problem] around…[then] together we recognised the issues…and discussed ideas on how to change it... It was a team effort, and I really enjoy discussing these topics in this way with others. It is so insightful to hear so many different views on the same topic [2].

Diverse networks influenced the development of ideas and the power to distribute them in various contexts [2]. In this way, diverse perspectives and relationships can enable collective creativity (ideas for solutions from many people thinking or acting together). These findings suggest that diversity of views/perspectives can enrich ideas for solutions and improve care and team working [2].

Workplace problems are best addressed through input from a wide range of individuals. The concept of participatory creativity, where solutions emerge through collective collaboration is considered essential for the best solution [14]. This approach draws on the unique experiences of individuals, creating a richer pool of ideas expressed and shaped through social interaction and shared actions. Whilst collective problem-solving often involves tensions, these discussions can help clarify which issues require negotiation whilst engaging with diverse perspectives, allowing for a more thorough examination of both problems and potential solutions [15, 16]. Some researchers advocate for co-designed tools and solutions, which are developed collaboratively to address real-world constraints more effectively [16].

For instance, co-designing a new hospital ward admission protocol can help resolve challenges experienced by different healthcare professionals, ensuring the final process better meets everyone's needs.

When exploring a broad range of perspectives on workplace problems, some individuals may resist or dismiss alternative viewpoints due to a reluctance to embrace new ways of working. This reaction is understandable in some ways, because some literature suggests that people often gravitate toward familiar and predictable routines [9]. However, in day-to-day healthcare practice, approaching problems from multiple angles and considering diverse solutions can lead to more informed decision-making and drive meaningful improvements [10].

Diverse Opportunities for Culture Change

Depending on the specific challenges in a workplace culture and the specific context of the team, there are several ways in which individuals can contribute towards culture-based change. The approaches discussed in the rest of this chapter are based on the principle of movement. It emphasises the active role each individual plays in recognising cultural norms and intentionally seeking ways to shift away from those that are problematic. Understanding and transforming workplace culture begins at the individual level, through the creation of opportunities that encourage different forms of movement. This includes theoretical movement, where individuals imagine and explore the potential outcomes of their own actions and those of others. It also involves empowering movement, which refers to using one's position or influence to support and uplift others, and social movement, where individuals make deliberate efforts to understand the roles and perspectives of colleagues, considering both their own and others' viewpoints. Finally, physical movement involves placing oneself in unfamiliar or uncomfortable environments to gain deeper insight into alternative perspectives or ways of working. Together, these forms of movement offer a framework for fostering cultural awareness and promoting meaningful change within healthcare settings.

Variability and heterogeneity in organisational culture is important [4]. Perceptions of workplace culture vary across roles and groups within organisations, and differences in perceptions about workplace culture and the varied ways of working among groups across an organisation can provide culture-based insight beneficial to inform change [17]. For instance, nursing teams on different wards may operate in distinct ways and face unique culture-related challenges. As a result, workplace culture issues might emerge in one department but not in another, even within the same organisation. In other parts of the same organisation or across different organisations, the nature of these problems can vary significantly. This is because culture-based issues are highly contextual and shaped by the local environment.

In my doctoral research, workplace behaviour was often shaped by a combination of policy, organisational culture (including micro-political dynamics) and broader political influences including recent independent inquiries into healthcare failures [2]. Participants were influenced by the priorities highlighted in national reports and professional publications and sought to respond to the issues they recognised. For example, one participant proposed ways to address inequalities in maternity care, whilst another offered suggestions for improving healthcare training. These examples show how external contexts, such as policy, literature and national reports, encouraged healthcare students to consider solutions to systemic problems. However, the case studies also revealed that many ideas were limited by a lack of opportunity and insufficient autonomy to act on them. Box 3.4 details a case study whereby a healthcare student wanted to make changes that improve care, but her ideas were constrained by lack of opportunity and lack of autonomy.

Box 3.4 Case Study Where a Lack of Opportunity to Share Ideas and a Lack of Autonomy Influences Workplace Culture
Ideas for improving care and healthcare education shared in my doctoral research included an idea to extend the length of postnatal maternity care support offered by midwives. The student recognised that some women needed support for a longer period of time than *usual*. She described how the senior and supervising midwife believed it was a good idea but also informed the student that the idea was not possible because the local hospital policy would not allow it. The local hospital policy stated that women should be discharged from maternity care at 10–14 days following the birth of their child, regardless of ongoing need or preference. The healthcare student accepted the norm of discharge at 10–14 days and did not take her idea any further.
This case demonstrates how,

- Established norms/policies can constrain healthcare improvement and innovation.
- The opportunity to share ideas from a range of individuals (including students) is important.
- That reduced autonomy to make individualised decisions in the workplace might lead to reduced quality of care and reduced contributions to improving care.

Opportunities for culture change are most beneficial when enacted in the local context because local social action is what sustains and creates the local culture, as connected with the broader organisational culture. In my doctoral research, local role modelling by senior staff, leaders and managers was found to influence social behaviour, sharing of ideas and workplace culture [2]. This included role modelling social behaviour in response to political matters; in other words, individuals should act within the local workplace culture (how it is expected that teams or groups work together including shared values, attitudes and goals). Cases illustrated that the modelled behaviours can either enable or constrain idea-sharing, innovation and improvements.

Introducing different ideas and perspectives can challenge established ways of working. These challenges may also disrupt existing power dynamics, particularly when those in positions of authority such as managers, leaders or senior professionals hold significant influence over which ideas are considered acceptable and who is allowed to present them [2]. Therefore, fostering culture change requires critically examining how power is distributed within teams and exploring ways to empower individuals to share their thoughts, concerns and ideas. This can happen through approaches that create movement. In healthcare settings, experienced professionals, educators, leaders, managers and supervisors typically hold more power to influence change. Their role gives them considerable sway over what becomes accepted within the workplace culture. This positions them to actively support and create opportunities for cultural transformation. However, culture change is not the responsibility of leaders alone, because every individual has the capacity to contribute. Box 3.5 includes a reflective task to help you explore how you can participate in and influence culture change within your own work environment through movement.

Box 3.5 Approaches That Use *Movement* to Contribute Towards Workplace Culture Change

Some individuals are *culture carriers* which means that some individuals can *carry a culture* substantially more than others [1]. They bring impact and a sense of community to a team and improve innovation and retention of talent. They see the social and culture-based problems surfacing through behaviours, and they challenge them [1]. For example, some individuals could be sensitive to social and cultural issues that surface as a conflict or communication issue between colleagues, or about tensions between different wards or departments.

Everyone has potential to be a *culture carrier* through building skills, by taking conscious steps towards recognising problems and bringing ideas for solutions.

1. Think about a social/culture-based workplace problem you are aware of as you consider the reflective points below.
    (a) *Theoretically imagining where a problem might lead and consciously thinking about how a problem that contributes to the working culture can aid in culture change.* Think about your problem from the perspectives of each of those involved. If it is a conflict between colleagues or a communication issue, think about how this might feel for those involved. They might feel frustrated from a lack of autonomy, or overwhelmed with too much work, or something else.

    How can you actively seek to understand different perspectives about the problem from those involved? Understanding the problem (not only from your own perspective) is key to making decisions about how problems can be addressed.

    How do you imagine the problem might influence the future behaviour of the team? Is this problem likely to become an embedded and established behaviour trait of the team? Where could this problem lead and what type of working culture does this problem create?

(b) *Empowering others can help to address culture-based problems* because solutions for culture-based problems are most likely to come from collective ideas. A manager or leader will not necessarily have the best solution to a problem, and so everybody will benefit from being open and hearing other ideas for solutions whilst acting to empower people to share ideas, concerns and questions. This supports a learning culture at all levels.

Thinking about the problem you identified at the start of this reflective task, what do you think the solution to the problem is and how can you share this?

How can *you* make sure that everyone can be heard? What opportunities could you create to hear other ideas, concerns and questions?

(c) *Theoretically imagining where a problem Social movement theory encourages us to examine how problems are experienced across different roles within a system.* Often, culture-based issues persist because individuals in positions of power respond in ways that unintentionally reinforce existing problems. These power holders can include a wide range of roles such as teachers, supervisors, shift leaders or more experienced staff members. The impact of an individual's behaviour on team culture is partly influenced by their position, particularly within hierarchical structures. Those with greater power have a significant role in shaping workplace culture, and their actions can either contribute towards positive change or perpetuate existing challenges.

Thinking about the workplace problem you have identified, in what way do leaders, managers and others involved enable the problem through their position within the team?

How can hierarchical or power influences enabling the behaviours be challenged? For example, if the behaviour is sustained by negative comments from shift leaders, what mechanisms or tools could help junior colleagues (or any colleague) to challenge the behaviour?

Would any information sharing, education or training be beneficial for the team?

(d) *Physically moving* can broaden our understanding of issues and possible solutions. We can also learn from different ways of working and draw on the strengths of other teams and colleagues.

Could you learn more about the problem by experiencing the problem from another physical/social position? For example, if you are a manager/leader, could you work on the ward to understand the perspectives of your ward team better?

Could you go and work in a different ward/department to understand problems from alternative role perspectives? Or actively seek to understand challenges on different wards/departments?

Being open to viewing and understanding problems from various perspectives is beneficial for solving problems and for innovation in healthcare. It supports *perspectival dialogue* which involves the conversing with a range of perspectives as important for enabling the sharing of ideas [12]. A workplace culture of limited diverse opportunities and limited openness to alternative perspectives constrains the sharing of ideas and innovative practice [2]. In contrast, engagement with diverse colleague perspectives and increased networking across wards, departments and organisations is enabling [2]. This aligns with theoretical perspectives that appreciate the diversity of ways a creative (idea-sharing) culture can be supported [18]. Diversity of information and experience for health professionals may challenge concepts and understanding because it can create dissonance that prompts growth, more creative and collective ideas and innovative solutions in response to challenges in the workplace. Isolated and insular healthcare teams are less well equipped for growth, innovation and change, whereas teams that expand their networks and perspectives about problems, whether across professional groups, wards, hospitals, nationally or internationally, are better equipped for change and growth.

Learning from Global Perspectives

Understanding global diversity in perspectives about issues can inform more diverse idea-sharing and can support an enriched learning culture with better understanding about issues and possible solutions.

The broader social and cultural context in which we live, beyond the boundaries of the workplace, shapes how we perceive problems, engage professionally and interact with one another. These external influences play a significant role in shaping our creative and idea-sharing capacities and collaborative behaviours to solve problems. Creative ideas and idea-sharing at work is not a singular or isolated phenomenon but rather distributed across multiple ecologies (systems and relationships between self and the wider context) [18]. These ecologies that encompass environments, partnerships, policies and processes can enable a wide range of creative expressions that span different cultures and boundaries [18]. In this way, multiple stakeholders can enrich ideas to solve problems and wider-reaching connections, including global connections, can offer new insight and improve collaborative efforts.

Building on this, creativity (thought process that leads to new ideas, idea-sharing and action) itself is a complex, multifaceted concept that is interpreted, valued and studied differently across cultures. This variation stems in part from its inherently value-laden nature, which carries moral dimensions that are socially, culturally or individually assigned [12]. Vlad Glăveanu, Associate Professor of Psychology in Norway, emphasises that creativity is complicated by the interplay of sociocultural, interconnected and interdependent factors that influence its development and expression [12]. The willingness to approach familiar situations in unfamiliar ways requires individuals to have an open mind to what alternative cultures and global perspectives can offer. It means that global connections and connections with unfamiliar cultures and ways of working can enrich ideas and problem-solving for culture-based problems locally.

In Western culture, the willingness to be creative and share ideas is often regarded as a deeply humanistic trait, closely tied to human potential, success, rationality and psychological wellbeing [9]. In contrast, other global cultures place greater emphasis on creativity and idea-sharing being about adaptability [19]. In Japanese culture, Satori is a concept that embodies personal devotion, continuous practice, focussed concentration and full mind-body engagement, ultimately leading to creative enlightenment and understanding [20]. In practice, idea-sharing in Western culture is considered part of reaching potential at work, whereas in other cultures, idea-sharing is viewed as reflective of full devotion and commitment to one's work. A notable point of convergence across cultural perspectives of creativity and idea-sharing is the shared recognition of the relationship between creativity and learning. Whether idea-sharing involves self-discovery, personal expression or the acquisition of knowledge that precedes innovation and creative action, it is deeply connected with learning and expression of learning. In essence, global understanding of idea-sharing is intertwined with learning and learning cultures. This suggests that creative thinking and idea-sharing are vital to fostering a culture of learning [21]. Some even suggest that creative thinking/doing and learning are inseparable [22] highlighting the importance of collaborative idea-sharing so that global ideas can inform global solutions and learning.

Summary

Are you moving or are you the status quo? Understanding how movement and diversity supports a positive learning culture in healthcare has been discussed in this chapter. Whilst stagnant culture resists change and innovation leading to a decline in staff wellbeing and performance, a learning culture prioritises learning, growth, sharing of ideas and innovation. Workplace culture can be analysed through reflective activities and tools, such as the Competing Values Framework [5]. Dominant culture-based practices in the workplace and understanding what the dominant features in your workplace are can aid ideas-sharing and in promoting a learning culture. Whether your organisation is more flexible and open to receiving ideas for improvement or more focussed on achieving competitive key performance indicators and other measures, there is always room for growth and innovation in healthcare and for individual professionals. Creating opportunities for culture change may include participating in a range of behaviours and actions that purposefully challenge you to think about problems from diverse perspectives and to reach collective solutions whilst overcoming social and cultural norms in the local context and hierarchical barriers. By drawing on diverse perspectives from other teams, industries or differing global perspectives and understanding, ideas to learn about and improve workplace culture is possible.

References

1. Grant A. Think again: the power of knowing what you don't know. London: Ebury Publishing; 2021.
2. Philp-Von Woyna L. A multi-case study to understand the ways in which sociocultural factors influence everyday creative contributions in healthcare and higher education by student midwives. Doctoral thesis. Staffordshire: Staffordshire University; 2025. Available from: https://eprints.staffs.ac.uk/8884/.
3. Lave J, Wenger E. Situated learning: legitimate peripheral participation. Cambridge: Cambridge University Press; 1991.
4. Tietschert M, Bahadurzada H, Kerrissey M. Revisiting organizational culture in healthcare: heterogeneity as a resource. Soc Sci Med. 2024;356:117165. https://doi.org/10.1016/j.socscimed.2024.117165. PMID: 39121526.
5. Quinn R, Rohrbaugh J. A spatial model of effectiveness criteria: toward a competing values approach to organizational analysis. Manag Sci. 1983;29:363–77. https://doi.org/10.1287/mnsc.29.3.363.
6. Sørensen JB. The strength of corporate culture and the reliability of firm performance. Adm Sci Q. 2002. https://doi.org/10.2307/3094891.
7. Corritore M, Goldberg A, Srivastava SB. Duality in diversity: how intrapersonal and interpersonal cultural heterogeneity relate to firm performance. Adm Sci Q. 2020;65(2):359–94. https://doi.org/10.1177/0001839219844175.
8. Baker R. A review of deaths of patients at Gosport War Memorial Hospital [Internet]. Gosport Review; 2003. Available from: https://www.gosportreview.nhs.uk.
9. Runco M. Creativity: research, development, and practice. London: Elsevier Science; 2023.
10. Livermore D. Driven by difference: how great companies fuel innovation through diversity. 1st ed. Nashville: AMACOM; 2016.
11. Edmondson A. The fearless organization: creating psychological safety in the workplace for learning, innovation, and growth. Hoboken: Wiley; 2018.
12. Glăveanu VP. A sociocultural theory of creativity: bridging the social, the material and the psychological. Rev Gen Psychol. 2020;24(4):335–54.
13. UK Civil Aviation Authority. Fatigue in air traffic management [Internet]. London: UK CAA. Available from: https://www.caa.co.uk/commercial-industry/airspace/air-traffic-management-and-air-navigational-services/fatigue-in-air-traffic-management/.
14. Hanchett Hanson M, Amato A, Durani A, Hoyden J, Koe S, Sheagren E, Yang Y. Creativity and improvised educations: case studies for understanding impact and implications. London: Routledge; 2021.
15. Hyrkkö S, Kajamaa A. Distributed creativity and expansive learning in a teacher training school's change laboratory. In: Lemmetty S, Collin K, Glăveanu V, Forsman P, editors. Creativity and learning: contexts, processes and support. London: Palgrave Macmillan; 2021.
16. Wong C, Kumpulainen K, Kajamaa A. Collaborative creativity among education professionals in a co-design workshop: a multidimensional analysis. Think Skills Creat. 2021;42:100953.
17. Zyphur MJ, Zammuto RF, Zhang Z. Multilevel latent polynomial regression for modeling (in)congruence across organizational groups: the case of organizational culture research. Organ Res Methods. 2015. https://doi.org/10.1177/1094428115588570.
18. Szabó T, Burnard P, Harris A, Fenyvesi K, Soundararaj G, Kangasvieri T. Multiple creativities put to work for creative ecologies in teacher professional learning: a vision and practice of everyday creativity. In: Lemmetty S, Collin K, Glăveanu V, Forsman P, editors. Creativity and learning: contexts, processes and support. London: Palgrave Macmillan; 2021.

19. Dobzhansky T. Mankind evolving. New Haven: Yale University Press; 1962.
20. Fouts A. Satori: toward a conceptual analysis. Buddh Christ Stud. 2004;24:101–16.
21. Lemmetty S, Collin K, Glăveanu V, Forsman P. Creativity and learning: contexts, processes and support. London: Palgrave Macmillan; 2021.
22. Craft A. Creativity in schools: tensions and dilemmas. London: Routledge; 2005.

Overworked, Overwhelmed, Fatigued and Burned Out: Reworking Wellbeing into Healthcare Practice

4

Introduction

The incidence of burnout, compassion fatigue and mental health problems is increasing among healthcare workers with consequences that impact individual wellbeing, teamwork and the quality and safety of patient care. Registered healthcare professionals are deciding to leave soon after qualifying with the most commonly cited reason being work-related exhaustion and burnout. Recent reports highlight that even the most basic needs of healthcare workers are not being met, such as adequate rest, food and hydration. In addition to this, the wider needs of individuals are reported as neglected. This chapter explores the individual and system level factors that can support healthcare worker wellbeing under seven key areas of focus. These are as follows:

(a) *Relationships*, including actions and interventions that promote positive workplace relationships and social connections that create a sense of belonging and foster compassion and respect for each other improve wellbeing.
(b) *Power* including how leaders and those in positions of power actively take steps to reduce power differences. This topic also includes hierarchical-based relationships across teams that increase psychological safety and wellbeing for all.
(c) *Autonomy* including providing opportunity for everyone to share ideas, express their opinions and concerns and ask questions as improving sense of wellbeing. Actions that increase autonomy, space for idea-sharing and improvement.
(d) *Openness* including teams that are open to new ideas, reward contributions and value a questioning attitude to promote a learning culture that is beneficial for wellbeing.
(e) *Collectivist action* because whilst blame cultures cause individuals to experience high levels of stress, collective problem-owning and collective problem-solving when challenges or errors occur fosters a learning culture beneficial for wellbeing.

L. Philp-von Woyna, *Unravelling Workplace Culture in Healthcare*, https://doi.org/10.1007/978-3-032-11771-7_4

(f) *Rewarding* individuals because personal opportunities for accomplishment, including opportunity for professional development and education, support a sense of wellbeing.
(g) *Meeting the basic needs* of individuals to create a culture where the people are at the centre. This includes supporting wider needs such as flexible working and practices where basic needs such as rest, hydration and food are always prioritised.

In this chapter, these themes and issues are explored as actionable strategies in further depth, drawing on media and professional reports. This includes reports of suicide among healthcare workers under significant work-related stress and reports where even the very basic needs of healthcare workers have been neglected in the workplace. Wellbeing is an increasingly important priority for individuals and organisations, and this chapter outlines what practical action can be taken to improve wellbeing for all.

No Water Allowed

In 2021, the UK's Nursing Times academic journal reported that nurses and midwives had restricted access to water whilst working on hospital wards [1]. The paper outlined the importance of staying hydrated whilst working hospital shifts along with the potential clinical implications of not doing so as impact on decision-making, memory, attention span, mood and tiredness [1]. The paper also challenges and debunks myths that suggest having fluid bottles on hospital wards presents a cross infection risk. Even small deficits in total body water can have a significant impact on performance and can cause sleepiness, headaches, impatience and apathy [2]. Two litres of water each day is required for normal cognitive performance, but some working environments may increase the water required to maintain normal cognitive function [2]. For instance, working in hospital ward environments often increases water loss meaning higher amounts of water intake are required because factors such as higher ambient temperatures for patient comfort and use of personal protective equipment (PPE) such as plastic aprons and gloves increase bodily fluid loss through perspiration [2]. Mild dehydration is not always recognised by individuals who are busy working, but relatively small body water losses equalling 1–2 kg may reduce cognitive function by 15–20% altering attitude to team tasks and in caring for patients [2].

The need for adequate rest, hydration and food to maintain cognitive performance and safety at work has been extensively studied in other industries. These core human needs have been studied as an aspect of *human factors* where literature consistently concludes that if these core needs are not met, then performance declines and errors increase [3]. Evidence does not support the practice of limiting water bottles on hospital wards to reduce infection risk. Therefore, the 2021 paper highlighting that water bottles were being restricted on hospital wards for fear of infection risk is an example of where normative practices and ingrained attitudes (towards basic needs) have created a *culture of acceptance*. People accept that water bottles will be restricted during their hospital shift, despite evidence suggesting this practice is not good for anyone, the individual staff, staff team and patient safety [3].

Developing strong skills in evidence analysis is essential for identifying practices that are not grounded in evidence and may be culturally ingrained. Recognising such behaviours allows for more informed decisions in shaping policy and guiding leadership. In healthcare, effective leadership plays a vital role in addressing these entrenched practices. One promising approach is compassionate leadership, which has the potential to uncover and address deeply rooted issues, ultimately reducing harm to both staff and patients [4]. Compassionate leadership involves *actively listening, empathising and responding to the needs of individuals* and the broader organisation. It is characterised by attentiveness to both fundamental human needs such as access to water, food, rest and legal rights as well as to broader psychological and emotional needs, including wellbeing, safety, belonging, identity and opportunities for personal growth through meaningful work. By fostering an environment where these needs are acknowledged and met, compassionate leadership can significantly enhance group wellbeing and organisational culture.

According to the UK's Health Foundation, one of the biggest challenges in healthcare relates to the wellbeing of staff [5]. The Health Foundation reported that nearly half of all healthcare workers felt unwell due to work-related stress in the last 12 months and 34% reported burnout [5]. Pressure on staff working in the UK health system is increasing as a combination of staff shortages, resource constriction, limited finances, high turnover of staff and increasing workloads collides [5]. These pressures are impacting the wellbeing of a range of healthcare workers. In global comparison, UK workers are among the worst affected with UK General Practitioners (GPs) reporting some of the highest levels of stress and lowest levels of job satisfaction compared to other high-income countries [5]. Pressures of the job are thought to be contributing towards many GPs and other health professionals saying they are considering leaving healthcare altogether [5]. The UK's Royal College of Nursing [RCN] analysed data trends of registered nurses and found that thousands of UK-educated nurses leave the profession shortly after qualifying [6]. Between 2021 and 2024, there was a 67% increase in the number of nurses leaving the profession within 5 years of registration, compared to figures reported in 2021 [6]. The UK's Nursing and Midwifery Council [NMC] suggests that the main reason nurses leave is due to *burnout and exhaustion* brought on by factors such as low staffing levels, increasing patient need and a lack of recognition from government through renumeration [7].

Promoting Workplace Wellbeing and Reducing Staff Burnout

There are a number of ways that individuals, healthcare organisations and wider society can support workplace wellbeing in healthcare to reduce exhaustion and burnout. Burnout is defined as a disease (with health impact) and a syndrome caused by chronic work-related stress that has not been successfully managed [8]. There have been recent efforts to understand the scale and scope of reported burnout among healthcare staff through inquiries such as one undertaken by Health and Care Select Committee in 2021 that conducted an inquiry focussed on workforce burnout and resilience in healthcare [9]. They concluded that burnout is widespread and common among healthcare workers in the UK and negatively impacts the mental health of individual staff, teamworking and the quality of care they provide for patients at work.

Creating opportunities for individuals to express emotions and share ideas or solutions can help reduce stress and support personal processing of challenging experiences ultimately contributing to a reduction in burnout symptoms [10]. Unpredictable and uncertain workplace environments may lead to emotional exhaustion, diminished feelings of personal accomplishment and symptoms commonly associated with burnout [10]. Literature also supports there is an association between uncertainty and adverse mental health outcomes. For instance, the COVID-19 pandemic underscored the impact of heightened uncertainty on the mental and physical wellbeing of healthcare professionals worldwide [11–13]. During this period, reports of burnout increased significantly, along with a higher likelihood of health professionals leaving the field and experiencing compassion fatigue [14–16].

Compassion fatigue, which shares many symptoms with burnout, is defined as emotional, physical and psychological exhaustion resulting from prolonged exposure to work-related stress and the suffering of others [17, 18]. Its effects are far-reaching, negatively impacting not only patient care but also the physical, emotional, social, spiritual and intellectual health of healthcare workers [19]. Factors thought to influence compassion fatigue include chronically high workloads and constant exposure to the suffering of others. Working in environments where demands for emotional investment are persistently high means there is greater need for factors that can aid processing of emotion and stress. Social connections at work and outside work are important for dealing with stress and change [10]. Less social contact and connections result in less opportunity to express and process workplace events and stresses with friends and colleagues [10]. This is significant because opportunities for self-expression with those we are socially connected with are associated with improved emotional processing and regulation, better mental health and improved wellbeing [20]. In addition, creative expression (which includes the bringing of ideas for healthcare improvement) is associated with increased cognitive flexibility, adaptable thinking, resilience and problem-solving [20]. This means that when healthcare workers have better social support, they are better able to process emotional and stressful work-related events and more resilient. In addition, opportunities for sharing ideas in the workplace and in social circles foster a sense of psychological wellbeing, support a sense of purpose in work and benefit psychological wellbeing [10]. The social aspects of the workplace are critical aspects that contribute towards the wellbeing of individual staff. What people do together at work, the informal and formal conversations and social meaning ascribed to such influence workplace culture. For instance, solving problems and driving improvements as a team (collaborative creative endeavours) not only builds community ties, interpersonal skills and social connectedness but also results in better solutions and improved wellbeing for everyone involved. In contrast, isolation (lack of meaningful relationships with colleagues and others) as well as chronic stress induced by high workloads, changing, unstable and unpredictable circumstances contributes towards increasing work-related burnout.

The incidence of burnout has increased significantly during and following the pandemic, and, consequently, the syndrome has come to be known as a *second* or *silent* pandemic [21]. Across society the impact of reduced social contact and quality of social connections during the pandemic is thought to be surfacing through increased mental health needs and a reduced sense of wellbeing. The World Health Organization (WHO) reports a 25% increase in the prevalence of anxiety and depression worldwide following the pandemic and the British Medical Association states that the restrictions designed to mitigate viral spread have influenced our mental health and wellbeing [22]. One in three adults reports a deterioration in mental health following the coronavirus pandemic [22], and whilst burnout is not a mental health illness in itself, it is strongly associated with development of a mental health illness [23]. The factors most associated with increased likelihood of burnout include high-stress levels, lack of social support, conflicts, unfair treatment, demanding workload, poor communication, lack of support from authority figures and a loss of sense of control and autonomy. Many of these factors are related to the *social workplace* whilst others are also related to aspects of the organisation and local leadership. As cases of burnout, compassion fatigue and mental health problems increase among healthcare workers, it is imperative that individuals, teams and organisations are aware of what actions can be taken to improve wellbeing. Box 4.1 provides an opportunity to reflect on the current practices in your workplace and begins to outline key areas that can promote and support staff wellbeing.

Box 4.1 Reflecting on Key Actions to Promote Staff Wellbeing and Reduce Burnout

(a) *Relationships* what actions and interventions promote positive workplace relationships and social connections? How do these practices create a sense of belonging and foster compassion and respect for each other that improves wellbeing?

(b) *Leaders and those in positions of power* can actively take steps to reduce power differences and hierarchy. What steps do leaders in your workplace take to reduce power differences and increase feelings of safety to speak up about issues?

(c) Is *autonomous practice* part of how you work? Do you have opportunities and the freedom to express your ideas, opinions, concerns and ask questions?

(d) Is *openness to new ideas*, a questioning attitude and learning from incidents part of how your team work together?

(e) Does your workplace assign blame for errors, or take *collective owner-ship* of errors? Does your workplace value collective problem-solving and learning?

(f) Are you rewarded for your accomplishments, provided with opportunity for professional development and further education?

(g) Are your basic needs met at work? Do you have adequate rest during the working day, adequate hydration and food? Are your wider needs met, such as flexible working?

In considering the reflective points above,

1. What does your workplace do well?
2. What areas require improvement in your workplace?
3. Write a strategy that actions some of the suggestions above. How do you think you could personally act, influence or support change through this strategy?

It Is Safe and *Important* to Express Yourself

The Centre for Creative Leadership suggest that psychological safety to be yourself and express yourself without fear of negative consequence is not only desirable but is essential for supporting a learning culture [24]. It enables the workforce to be better equipped to prevent failures and increases team resilience and problem solving. Creating an environment that is psychologically safe means ensuring that every team member feels safe to take interpersonal risks, like speaking up with ideas, questions, concerns or mistakes, without experiencing negative repercussions. Creating psychological safety at work is not about being nice to each other all the time, but it is about having the freedom and autonomy to share ideas and thoughts, to openly challenge the status quo, give feedback to each other and work through disagreements that arise together [24]. The individual contributions of every worker are important for creating a safer workplace [25]. One individual could be the person who provides a single piece of feedback or an opinion that is the 'mission critical' component of a positive change [25]. Psychological safety at work is about ensuring there is an environment where individual views can be shared with confidence those views will be valued [25]. Whilst work environments will often experience points of conflict, differing views and disagreements, a psychologically safe environment is one where these conflicts and differing views will be harnessed and understood so that, collectively, better solutions can be found [25].

Individuals all have unique, intrinsic motivating reasons for sharing thoughts and ideas [26]. These intrinsic reasons might include sharing our thoughts or ideas for our own personal enjoyment or satisfaction it brings us, for achieving a sense of purpose and meaning or because we are passionate about particular topics and wish to express that [26]. These intrinsic factors are different to the extrinsic factors (external factors) that may influence why we share thoughts and ideas at work. Extrinsic motivating factors to share ideas and thoughts might include receiving praise, receiving recognition in a social environment from peers or seniors or receiving rewards. Whilst intrinsic and extrinsic factors both contribute towards creating a psychologically safe working culture, intrinsic factors are often neglected in organisational strategies to improve workplace culture but deserve increased focus. This is because humanistic theory and research suggests that as humans we have a *need* for personal expression. Expressing oneself (creative expression) is imperative for self-actualisation (achieving one's potential) and cannot be separated from psychological health and wellbeing [27]. This means that being our best selves involves creatively expressing (sharing) ideas, thoughts and actions as part of living a fulfilled life with good psychological health and wellbeing. In a workplace context, these theoretical beliefs would suggest that a workplace that enables individual expression of ideas promotes psychological wellbeing, satisfaction and fulfilment. Participation in idea-sharing activities has been strongly linked to positive mental health, wellbeing and job satisfaction [10, 20, 28]. Furthermore, the ability to express oneself—whether through sharing ideas or engaging in creative and expressive activities—plays a significant role in helping individuals process and respond to everyday stressors, effectively contributing to the creation of a sense of wellbeing [28].

At times, the social environment can inhibit creative expression, as individuals may feel discouraged from sharing their true thoughts or proposing solutions due to fear of judgment or lack of confidence [29, 30]. For leaders, managers and decision-makers in healthcare, cultivating curiosity about others' perspectives and creating safe spaces for open dialogue can enhance wellbeing, foster problem-solving and positively influence organisational culture [31, 32]. This approach promotes a culture that values individuals' thoughts and feelings and actively seeks out their ideas, challenges and contributions. Developing the confidence to be oneself regardless of others' opinions is essential for psychological wellbeing [27]. Similarly, when individuals feel free to express their thoughts and ideas, they often experience improved wellbeing and greater job satisfaction and are more likely to contribute meaningfully to team efforts [33, 34]. The concept of perceived personal freedom, which includes autonomy and the ability to express oneself, is linked to enhanced emotional and mental health, as well as improved collaboration and creativity within teams [33, 34]. The flourishing and wellbeing of healthcare professionals are shaped by three key factors: autonomy, a sense of belonging and opportunities to contribute [31, 32]. Meeting these needs can transform individuals' work experiences and significantly improve the safety and quality of care they deliver.

Box 4.2 focusses on a reflective task about workplace actions/practices that promote psychological wellbeing and expression. Here you can reflect on the opportunities and constraints you face in bringing your opinions and ideas to the workplace.

Box 4.2 Reflect on Workplace Opportunities and Barriers to Share Your Ideas and Express Your Opinions

It is important to share your thoughts, ideas and opinions at work about the challenges and problems you encounter because it contributes towards your wellbeing, job satisfaction, effective teamworking and patient safety.

1. *Think about the key challenges you face at work.* It may include problems such as staffing shortages, too many tasks, not enough resource, time constraints, lack of opportunity for professional growth or something else.
2. What do you think are the possible ways to share ideas to make a difference in this area? What are the barriers to sharing your idea for solving the problem? The table below may prompt you to think about how to overcome barriers and/or create opportunities to act.

Creating opportunities	Overcoming barriers
Hierarchical opportunities Can you share your idea with people in roles at different levels of hierarchy?	*Power differences as a barrier* What tools/models/existing processes could you use to approach those with more power about your idea?
Peer opportunities What opportunities could you create for sharing your ideas with your peers?	*Lack of space to share ideas/opinions* How could you create a space?
Policy opportunities Could your idea feed into policy development?	*Rigid, goal orientated processes* Do some rigid, goal orientated processes need challenging?
National opportunities Could you share your ideas with peers/professionals outside your organisation?	*Lack of research about solutions* Could you contribute towards research, publications or forums to highlight the lack of evidence?
Educational opportunities Could you engage in educational opportunities or be part of educating others?	*Social opportunities* How can you reach out and build positive relationships with others around you that enable ideas?

3. What are the key actions you can take forward to share an idea to address a problem you have identified?

Conversations Matter for Wellbeing

To truly understand an organization's culture, just listen to the conversations. How people interact with one another—in the hallways, in conference rooms, in one-on-ones, even in informal chats by the coffee maker—it is the truest indicator of a company's culture…and investments in strengthening the quality of conversations across the organization…will quite literally…lead to a better culture [24].

Relationships and conversations between colleagues should not be underestimated for improving individual wellbeing and organisational culture and solving problems that arise in the workplace. Conversations are imperative to shape collective ideas and action, and the wide-reaching benefits of social connection have been discussed as important individual psychological wellbeing. However, in addition to individual wellbeing benefits, sharing opinions and ideas also supports team purpose.

Ideas and opinions begin with the individual, but the *community or network* influences whether a particular idea or opinion gathers momentum in development, direction and action [35]. This understanding is supported by a theory called the *network of enterprise* which maps the outline of a person's idea development suggesting it is a process which is developed over time, through building new perspectives (new points of view) in networked (social) positions, within systems (the healthcare system) [35]. It means that individuals may think of ways to solve problems in healthcare, but the wider social-professional group help those ideas to develop, gain momentum in action and, eventually, facilitate a solution.

In healthcare, addressing complex challenges often requires collaborative, group-developed solutions; however, the initial ideas that drive these solutions typically originate from individual perspectives and insights. This highlights the importance of personal opinions and ideas, not only for enhancing one's own sense of purpose and wellbeing but also for strengthening teamwork and improving patient care [35]. Wallace and Gruber [35] explored this concept through a series of case studies on influential thinkers, including Charles Darwin. Their analysis revealed that Darwin's groundbreaking ideas evolved over time through dialogue and interaction with his social network, including conversations that involved disagreement and error. They emphasised that social factors can either enable or inhibit the sharing of ideas and opinions. In Darwin's case, his initial reluctance to share his work stemmed from fear of public rejection, and it took many years before he felt confident enough to present his theories [35]. Individuals might fear how ideas or opinions might be received, and this may prevent them from sharing how they think and feel about challenges and issues in healthcare [10]. Fear of public rejection is rooted in group culture and the expectations and beliefs of a group [36]. Social groups that hold strong, established views on particular topics or practices can create an environment where individuals feel fearful about challenging those norms. Deeply ingrained practices are often difficult to question, as they may discourage alternative thinking and reduce confidence in those who wish to work differently. Individuals may anticipate that their ideas will be dismissed, and often, this proves true [36]. However, increasing awareness of how our own perspectives may differ from those around us, alongside a deeper understanding of the challenges involved in shifting workplace culture, can help foster more open and constructive conversations. These conversations have the potential to enhance wellbeing and support meaningful change [10].

Box 4.3 offers an opportunity to explore this topic further through personal reflection.

Box 4.3 Conversations to Value Your Own and Other Opinions and Ideas

1. Have you ever thought 'there is no point sharing my opinion on that because I know I won't be heard, and my views won't be taken seriously'? These thoughts often provide insight into problematic ingrained practices and opinions of groups that could provide insight into areas of culture most in need of change. Sharing your thoughts and opinions even when you suspect they may not be supported can be both empowering and beneficial for your wellbeing. It also plays a vital role in fostering a positive workplace culture by helping to identify and address underlying issues. *Speaking up* challenges the status quo and shifts the narrative from passive acceptance of dominant, potentially problematic norms to active engagement in cultural change. Whilst initial attempts to voice your ideas may be met with resistance, dismissal or lack of recognition, it is important to understand that such reactions often stem from entrenched cultural behaviours. Choosing to express your views despite these challenges not only supports your own psychological wellbeing but also encourages others to do the same. Over time, this can influence the attitudes and behaviours of those around you, contributing to a more open, inclusive and reflective workplace environment.

   Revisit Box 3.5 to understand how you can start conversations that influence change and mean your opinion, idea and views are heard.

2. Think of a time when you have been taken by surprise at another person's opinion about a problem at work.

   (a) How did you react? What did you say or do?

   (b) Did you shut down their opinion? (tell them that's not how it is/how it happened)

   You may have encountered situations where someone's interpretation of a work-related issue differs significantly from your own. In such moments, especially when holding a position of influence, it can be tempting to dismiss opposing views in favour of your own or the dominant perspective of the group. However, doing so can discourage others from sharing their opinions in the future and contributes to the persistence of entrenched, culture-based issues.

   When individuals feel silenced or unsupported, it reinforces a workplace culture that resists change. By contrast, encouraging diverse viewpoints even when they challenge the norm can foster psychological safety, promote open dialogue and support cultural transformation. Recognising and respecting differing opinions is essential for building a more inclusive and reflective work environment.

3. Thinking about how the person took you by surprise, what conversations could you start to better understand their views and think about how your own and their opinion might both contribute towards a positive workplace?

Conversations with others matter for creating a workplace where individuals feel valued, like they belong and for a sense of wellbeing. Making intentional efforts to promote dialogue between yourself and others at work that build skills in giving and receiving constructive feedback that is respectful can help promote individual wellbeing and support a group learning culture [37].

Healthcare organisations and professionals can take proactive steps to create space for meaningful team dialogue. This may involve developing skills around giving and receiving feedback and creating environments where colleagues feel safe to voice unspoken concerns. Such open communication can lead to more comprehensive and collaborative problem-solving.

Box 4.4 outlines practical opportunities for building skills in team dialogue and feedback, offering guidance on how to foster more inclusive and reflective conversations within healthcare teams.

Box 4.4 Opportunities for Improving Workplace Dialogue

There are many actions and strategies that individuals and organisations can support to improve team dialogue/conversation. Some potential strategies are described as follows:

1. *Create space for conversations*

   Creating space for conversations through interventions such as the *cup of coffee* approach can provide opportunities for problems and unprofessional social behaviours to be addressed early [38, 39]. The *cup of coffee* approach involves an informal conversation between peers. Typically, peers will have received training to lead a private, nonjudgmental conversation focussed on a concerning behaviour. The goal is to promote individual accountability, encourage reflection and open communication and positive behavioural change. It is an example of an approach to promote meaningful dialogue between colleagues that supports a learning culture.

   Reflect

   Can you think of other opportunities for meaningful dialogue among your team?

2. *Do more than active listening*

   Listening to workplace tensions or conflicts can inform strategies for improving team conversations. Better conversation skills in times of conflict or tension can be learned, and paying attention by listening is crucial to inform conversation [24]. There are multiple layers to group communication, each offering valuable insights that can benefit individuals who take the time to listen and reflect.

   Reflect

   (a) Think about a recent meeting or interaction that you had at work where a disagreement or tension arose.

   (b) Reflect on the layers of communication you observed.

Layer 1: Factual Content—This is typically the primary focus of communication. It involves the actual information being shared. What was said, reported or described?

Layer 2: Values and Priorities—This layer reflects the underlying values, beliefs and priorities that the communicator brings to the conversation. It helps reveal what matters most to them and why they are communicating in a particular way. What values or priorities do you think were being communicated?

Layer 3: Emotions—This final layer involves the emotional tone or feelings expressed during the conversation. Recognising the emotions behind the words can deepen understanding and improve interpersonal connection. What emotions do you think each person was bringing to the conversation?

Thinking about communication problems in several layers can uncover where communication issues really exist and the underlying reasons. This may be a clash of beliefs about the facts, a clash of values/professional judgement about what is most important/priorities or a clash of emotions. By reflecting on conflict or tensions, individuals can uncover where objections, reservations and barriers exist.

(c) Thinking about the meeting or interaction where you observed a tension or disagreement, was it a factual disagreement? A difference in values or priorities? Or a difference in emotions about an issue?

More than active listening can help you to recognise what your colleagues value, believe and feel at work and help you to be curious and better understand issues.

3. *Be curious and ask questions*

Asking questions in conversation is an art and science that can aid understanding about issues [24]. Listening to tensions or conflicts and being curious about what is happening can aid deeper insight into issues. For example, if tension arises over who should lead a particular clinical task, active listening may reveal underlying concerns—such as reservations about a colleague's suitability or confusion over task responsibilities. In such cases, asking open, nondirective questions can help uncover the root of the issue. This approach encourages honest dialogue, allowing team members to express concerns that might otherwise remain hidden, and supports more thoughtful, collaborative problem-solving.

(a) Think about the conflict or tension you have identified. What nondirective questions could you ask to uncover a deeper understanding of the tension/conflict?

4. *Balance 'challenge' and 'support' in conversation*

When we encounter tension or conflict in the workplace, it is natural to challenge the views or perspectives of our colleagues. However, effective communication requires that challenge be balanced with support.

Constructive disagreement involves expressing differing opinions whilst still valuing the other person's perspective. If individuals are challenged without feeling supported, it can lead to defensiveness and discourage them from sharing ideas or opinions in the future. Striking a balance between challenge and support helps build trust, encourages open dialogue and contributes to a healthier, more inclusive workplace culture.

A. Thinking about the example of tension or conflict you have identified, how would you challenge and support all viewpoints involved?

5. *Have honest and constructive conversations*

Have you ever skirted around the truth to avoid having a difficult conversation? We often learn to keep problems and opinions to ourselves and react to those in higher positions of power than us with facts and objectiveness [24]. However, this sometimes results in missed opportunities to provide feedback or to have constructive conversations with our colleagues about tasks, issues or events.

Constructive conversation is important, and it prioritises developing mutual understanding through striving to better understand others' views whilst feeling that others are striving to better understand yours [37, 40]. Constructive conversations are more likely to enable learning because the focus shifts to your own understanding of issues and efforts to understand others. In doing so, you can enrich your own perspective or worldview, clarify differences, discover common ground or help collaborative ideas and action (or even create the possibility of future collaborative action that may have previously seemed impossible). Whilst challenging others can promote defensiveness and breakdown of relationships, aiming to understand others can better inform constructive ways to move forward together and can strengthen relationships [40].

6. *Agree actions and accountability in conversation*

Conservations with purpose and clear, agreed actions that value all involved can help to support positive change [37]. Setting and agreeing clear actions can ensure that individuals do not feel overwhelmed but empowered to take steps towards positive change.

(a) Thinking about the example of conflict or tension you identified, how did the conversation end? Did any team members become defensive?

(b) How do you think you could value each perspective and agree joint actions in a similar circumstance in the future?

Organisations that Promote Holistic Individual Wellbeing

Organisations and those in leadership and management positions heavily influence workplace culture and the wellbeing of workers. There are several actions that organisational leaders and organisations can do to promote individual wellbeing.

These include factors such as actively supporting flexible working, supporting a learning culture, psychologically safe workplaces, group ownership of problems, group problem-solving and investing in people whilst recognising their achievement and offering fair working conditions and renumeration. Here each of these actions to support wellbeing are explored further.

Supporting Flexible Working

The Working Families Index report found that the healthcare industry was the most inflexible employing industry in the UK in 2025 [41]. All other employing industries in the UK, including those such as marketing, banking, retail and education, offered more flexible working options for their employees compared to healthcare. Flexible working is an arrangement which supports an individual to have greater choice in when, where and how they work [42]. It can include deciding on fixed working hours and shifts that individuals wish to work or a change in the location or type of work. It enables people to have better predictability and control over work schedules, and evidence suggests that it can be incredibly powerful in promoting employee wellbeing. Flexible work can reduce stress, improve health and save employers money [43, 44]. In addition, supporting flexible working in healthcare positively impacts patient safety by enhancing staff wellbeing, reducing staff burnout and improving staff retention [42]. Flexible working can ultimately lead to a more sustainable and responsive healthcare system.

In 2023, the British Medical Journal (BMJ) hosted a roundtable discussion examining the NHS's institutional intolerance towards flexible working in the UK [45]. Participants at the round table meeting discussed the damaging effect this is having on staff skills, retention and patient safety. Key contributors at the roundtable meeting were Rachel Hutchings, a fellow of the Nuffield Trust and co-author of the Future Proof report [46] which examined flexible working challenges for surgeons and Farzana Hussain, a general practitioner based in London, UK. Rachel identified that a *negative workplace culture* towards surgeons who worked part-time was largely to blame, and Farzana explained how the *workplace culture* made people afraid to say they needed an amendment or change in work pattern. Farzana expressed that people *don't feel safe to say* what flexible working patterns they need and suggested it has a direct negative impact on patient care. In the Future Proof report, workplace culture was noted as a consistent challenge and barrier to flexible working [46]. The report also detailed how the practical organisation of care, services and training as well as lack of support for employees with health conditions or caring responsibilities also contributes towards poor organisational support for flexible working. The BMJ concluded that flexible working is still too often inflexible in UK healthcare, and inflexible work is linked to patient safety concerns reporting on six strategies that could tackle it [45].

1. *Proactive support*—Employers should actively promote flexible working making employees aware of their options. A culture that positively welcomes flexible working choice can be beneficial [46].

2. *Lessons from primary care*—Primary care services in the UK offer more flexibility than other specialties and adjust service provision to facilitate the flexible working of staff. This includes examples of changing patient service times to earlier or later schedules and at the weekend to meet staff childcare responsibilities and other commitments outside of work. Many staff members may decide to leave their jobs if it does not fit around their caring responsibilities [45].

3. *Better planning*—There is a fear among leaders in healthcare that if the *floodgates* are opened for flexible working for all, then there will be more workforce staffing problems, but evidence suggests that it is unlikely [45]. The most likely outcome would be a requirement for better planning, and a more agile workforce can bring unexpected and different benefits [45].

4. *Role modelling*—It is important to employ senior people who work flexibly. They role model that flexible working is welcome and encouraged.

5. *Embrace the challenge*—Changing and adapting services and working collaboratively to support flexible working with 24-hour service needs may be difficult, but it is not impossible and embracing the challenge means more staff will choose to stay with their current employer [45].

6. *Think about patients*—Patients should be aware of realistic challenges for some aspects of care, such as models of care that aim to provide continuity of care. Flexible working can bring additional challenges in these areas, and patients should be involved in making decisions and their options.

Through organisational level commitment to removing the barriers for flexible working, the wellbeing of staff can be improved. Rather than viewing flexible working as not possible, organisations that prioritise the wellbeing of staff may improve patient care, safety, staff retention and innovation.

Supporting a Learning Culture, Physical and Psychological Safety

The workplace needs to attract and retain health and care workers by providing decent working conditions and fair remuneration and safeguarding worker rights [47]. This means providing healthcare workers with a safe, healthy, supportive and dignified conditions of work. At the basic level, physical spaces for staff changing areas, toilets, areas for rest, breastfeeding and expressing/storing breastmilk and access to water and food are required. Time is needed for adequate rest, hydration and to eat. At the start of this chapter, reference was made to recent reports of incidents even the most basic of needs is not met in the healthcare workplace [1]. When these basic needs are not met, errors are more likely and so meeting basic needs is imperative for providing safe patient care [2]. Whilst healthcare is a complex system and errors inevitably happen, steps can be taken to ensure that errors are minimised whilst also supporting the wellbeing of staff.

It is impossible to create a completely error-free healthcare system, and when errors do occur, it is important learn from them and recognise that it is often the surfacing of *system errors* through human acts [48]. Despite this, the culture of healthcare organisations can mean individuals are often blamed for errors. A blame culture assigns blame to the individual rather than trying to understand the various processes in the system that led to the individual making the fault [48]. A blame culture has a significant psychological impact on those working in healthcare, particularly those providing direct care. For example, a recent system failure in a London hospital led a young nurse to taking her own life when she feared humiliation and blame [48]. Sadly, this is not an isolated case with the General Medical Council conducting a review that found at least 28 suicides as linked to fitness-to-practice investigations [49]. These cases illustrate (but do not fully represent) the scale of suffering and stress that can be caused by *investigations* that assign blame to individual healthcare workers who may become the *victims of system failures.*

Steps are underway to address the blame culture problem in UK healthcare. Initiatives led by NHS England set out the principles under a Patient Safety Incident Response Framework (PSIRF) specification [50]. They state that a series of mindset principles should guide investigations into patient safety concerns. These principles include the following:

1. *Focus on the improvement* from incidents, not the process of investigating incidents.
2. *Avoiding the blame of individuals* because it limits insight into what went wrong. Instead, increased focus on how the system (team, organisation factors) may have contributed towards the incident will provide better insight into what can be learned.
3. *Learning is essential* to inform improvements. At times, no wrongs have occurred, but rather there is just a better way that has come to light through learning from an incident.
4. *Collaboration is key.*
5. *Psychological safety* is essential to learn from incidents because a climate of openness to different perspectives, team discussion around weaknesses and a willingness to suggest ideas for solutions aids improvement efforts.
6. *Leaders need to be curious* about why incidents occurred, not judgmental towards individuals.

Despite attempts to support a learning culture in healthcare, an NHS staff survey published in 2024 shows no significant change from recent years [51]. Questions specifically related to reporting incidents, clinical safety and *speaking up* about patient safety issues have not changed with a dominant blame culture remaining a recurring theme echoed across many different inquiries. For example, culture was found to contribute towards major patient safety concerns at East Kent NHS [52], Shrewsbury and Telford Hospitals NHS [53] and Mid-Staffordshire NHS [54]. Blame cultures encourage individuals to cover up problems for fear of retribution which can explain why *team and group-owned approache*s to learning from incidents and solving problems are so desperately needed.

Supporting Group Ownership of Problems and Group Problem-Solving

Group problem-solving is an essential element of supporting a learning culture that is often overlooked [10]. Sharing ideas and learning and acting together to improve healthcare greatly relies on *team-ownership and team problem-solving* which is only possible with a foundation of positive team relationships [10]. A workplace culture that fosters *group* ownership of challenges, errors and problems and engages everyone in strategies that bring diverse individual perspectives together to solve problems better supports the group learning culture [10]. Group ownership of problems and group problem-solving contributes towards building psychological safety, improved solutions and improved individual wellbeing [10]. This does not mean that individuals cannot be held accountable for deliberate or neglectful action but focusses on an understanding that challenges and problems most frequently come about because of factors related to the functioning of healthcare as a system. This includes how the organisation functions and operates and how individuals work together in teams, not as isolated individuals [10]. Ways to promote group ownership and problem solving may include improved focus and activity through the following:

- Improved transparency and communication about errors and challenges in organisations
- Open and candid conversations about challenges or errors as 'group problems' with focus on the ways that a similar error could be prevented in the future
- Ensuring a learning-focussed culture is prioritised over a blame-focussed culture.

Whether groups are successful in problem-solving together relies heavily on their relationships with each other but also the local social and micro-political environment and, more broadly, the economic and political events [55]. These factors come together and influence how well social groups can function and work together effectively and positively. Understanding that we are part of a bigger system where we are influenced by the power of others and the wider social, political and economic factors can aid understanding about why some group culture problems are difficult to overcome.

There are often tensions between the type of changes we want to see as individuals at work and what is possible for an individual (alone) to change within a system. However, understanding that we can be *active participants* in our world is important to aid recognition that the group culture is a culmination of individual thought and action [10, 55]. The term *individual agency* describes the action of individuals (to act/ be an agent) as part of a wider group. Collectively, individual agency alters group functioning and group culture and improves individual wellbeing.

Exercising individual agency is closely linked to emotional wellbeing, a sense of purpose and the unique knowledge each person contributes to their team [35]. Sharing ideas within a team is a key developmental milestone, essential for professional growth and learning [27]. In healthcare settings, this growth involves experimenting and engaging within the social and professional dynamics of the team [10].

To support this, individuals need opportunities to understand how their workplace functions, its strengths, challenges and cultural norms whilst also feeling safe to express their own ideas and perspectives. Contributing ideas in the healthcare workplace not only enhances individual wellbeing but also fosters a culture of learning, drives innovation and supports improvements in patient safety and quality of care [56].

Supporting Individual Accomplishment, Recognition and Role Progression

Individual opportunities to develop understanding about healthcare issues, challenges and strengths, particularly opportunities focussed on improving understanding about workplace culture, can support sharing ideas and improvements in healthcare [10]. Supporting individual development opportunities is not just about individual growth and wellbeing but also an investment in the wellbeing and effectiveness of teams and organisations. This is because the individual is inextricably and interdependently related to the workplace social climate and its working culture (norms). Organisations often represent and reflect the collective values and beliefs of the individual people who work in the organisation [57]. Therefore, investment in individuals and their development translates to investment in organisations, teams and the care they provide.

Despite clear evidence that education, training and development opportunities can improve the safety and retention of healthcare staff [42], there remains underinvestment or unclear investment in education beyond initial training for healthcare staff in the UK. This limits individual aspiration and accomplishment and in turn can limit job satisfaction and retention. The NHS Long-Term Workforce Plan [58] aims to address some of these issues through a comprehensive strategy to improve investment in education, retention of staff and reforming delivery of healthcare. The plan was written to address critical staffing challenges in healthcare and to ensure the NHS has the workforce it needs over the next 15 years. It sets out plans to increase the number of trainee nurses, doctors and other staff, improve wellbeing at work and alter how healthcare is delivered and distributed across acute and primary care [58]. However, the plan has received some criticism for overfocussing on long-term investment in training (which will take years to make a difference) whilst neglecting the issues that are problematic in healthcare today. The plan overlooks healthcare pay disputes and working conditions, bottlenecks in career development and education opportunities for individuals and lacks clarity about how delivery of care and healthcare roles may change over time.

Several strategies and approaches need to support opportunities for individual development and acquiring of new skills with recognition and reward. Recognition and reward may include role progression and renumeration, with the WHO Global Strategy on Human Resources for Health (2016–2030) explicitly calling for government and policymakers to ensure there are equal opportunities for career progression as well as recognition and rewards for skill development [59]. They suggest that emphasis should be placed on the need for supportive working conditions that allow health and care workers to grow professionally and which encourages investment in workforce development.

Summary

Wellbeing for individuals is a priority which if properly addressed has the potential to alter the number of issues and errors occurring in healthcare and the learning that can happen after incidents occur. In this chapter, a range of ways that the wellbeing of healthcare workers can be supported has been covered. This has included thinking about how the individual needs of staff are met by creating a workplace culture that prioritises staff rest, hydration and breaks with meals, as well as how the wider needs of staff are met, including work schedules, patterns and opportunities for personal and professional development. Strategies and reflective tasks have enabled you to think about the ways that you can improve wellbeing at work for yourself, but also the issues that need support from leaders and organisations. This helped you identify where workplace culture problems exist related to your own and your team's wellbeing needs. Building social connections, compassion for each other at work, group ownership of incidents and problems, group problem-solving and group learning have been central to much of the discussion.

References

1. Castella T. Banning drinking water for staff on wards "misguided", warns union. Nurs Times [Internet]. 2021. Available from: https://www.nursingtimes.net.
2. Brennan PA, Oeppen RS. The role of human factors in improving patient safety. Trends Urol Mens Health. 2022;13(3):30–3. https://doi.org/10.1002/tre.858.
3. Riebl SK, Davy BM. The hydration equation: update on water balance and cognitive performance. ACSMs Health Fit J. 2013;17:21–8.
4. Civility Saves Lives. Understanding the impact of rudeness on patient care and outcomes [Internet]. Civility Saves Lives. Available from: https://www.civilitysaveslives.com/.
5. Dunn P, Ewbank L, Alderwick H. Nine major challenges facing health and care in England. London: The Health Foundation; 2023. Available from: https://www.health.org.uk/reports-and-analysis/briefings/nine-major-challenges-facing-health-and-care-in-england.
6. Royal College of Nursing. Huge increase in nurses quitting early in 'perfect storm' for patient care, as RCN warns NHS reforms at risk [Internet]. London: RCN; 2024. Available from: https://www.rcn.org.uk/news-and-events/press-releases.
7. Nursing and Midwifery Council. Professionals who left the NMC register in 2024/2025 [Internet]. London: NMC; 2025. Available from: https://www.nmc.org.uk.
8. World Health Organization. Global health and care worker compact: technical guidance compilation [Internet]. Geneva: WHO; 2022. Available from: https://www.who.int/publications/i/item/9789240073852.
9. Health and Social Care Committee. Workforce burnout and resilience in the NHS and social care [Internet]. London: UK Parliament; 2021. Available from: https://committees.parliament.uk.
10. Philp-Von Woyna L. A multi-case study to understand the ways in which sociocultural factors influence everyday creative contributions in healthcare and higher education by student mid-

wives. Doctoral thesis. Staffordshire: Staffordshire University; 2025. Available from: https://eprints.staffs.ac.uk/8884/.

11. Hasheminejad N, Amirmahani M, Tahernejad S, Reza H, Nik T. Evaluation of work ability index and its association with job stress and musculoskeletal disorders among midwives during the Covid-19 pandemic. Med Lav. 2022;113(4):e2022031. https://doi.org/10.23749/mdl.v113i4.12834.

12. Jasiński AM, Derbis R, Walczak R. Workload, job satisfaction and occupational stress in Polish midwives before and during the COVID-19 pandemic. Med Pr. 2021;72(6):623–32. https://doi.org/10.13075/mp.5893.01149.

13. Li S, Chai R, Wang Y, Wang J, Dong X, Xu H, et al. A survey of mental health status of obstetric nurses during the novel coronavirus pneumonia pandemic. Medicine (Baltimore). 2021;100(52):e28070. https://doi.org/10.1097/md.0000000000028070.

14. Woeber K, Vanderlaan J, Long MH, Steinbach S, Dunn JL, Bouchard ME. Midwifery autonomy and employment changes during the early COVID-19 pandemic. J Midwifery Womens Health. 2022;67(5):608–17. https://doi.org/10.1111/jmwh.13400.

15. Aydin Dogan R, Huseyinoglu S, Yazici S. Compassion fatigue and moral sensitivity in midwives in COVID-19. Nurs Ethics. 2023;30(6):776–88. https://doi.org/10.1177/09697330221146224.

16. Ahmadi S, Maleki A. The relationship between burnout and intention to leave work among midwives: the long-lasting impacts of COVID-19. J Healthc Eng. 2022:8608732. https://doi.org/10.1155/2022/8608732.

17. Duarte J, Pinto-Gouveia J, Cruz B. Relationships between nurses' empathy, self-compassion and dimensions of professional quality of life: a cross-sectional study. Int J Nurs Stud. 2016;60:1–11. https://doi.org/10.1016/j.ijnurstu.2016.02.015.

18. Peters E. Compassion fatigue in nursing: a concept analysis. Nurs Forum. 2018;53(4):466–80. https://doi.org/10.1111/nuf.12274.

19. Abernathy S, Martin R. Reducing compassion fatigue with self-care and mindfulness. Nurs Crit Care [Internet]. 2019;14(5):38–44. Available from: https://www.researchgate.net/publication/335648245.

20. Jean-Berluche D. Creative expression and mental health. J Creat. 2024;34(2):100083. https://doi.org/10.1016/j.yjoc.2024.100083.

21. Medina-Dominguez F, Sanchez-Segura MI, de Amescua-Seco A, Dugarte-Peña GL, Villalba Arranz S. Agile Delphi methodology: a case study on how technology impacts burnout syndrome in the post-pandemic era. Front Public Health. 2023;10:1085987.

22. British Medical Association. The impact of the pandemic on population health and health inequalities [Internet]. London: BMA; 2024. Available from: https://www.bma.org.uk.

23. Maddock A. The relationships between stress, burnout, mental health and well-being in social workers. Br J Soc Work. 2023;54(2):668–86. https://doi.org/10.1093/bjsw/bcad232.

24. Center for Creative Leadership. Better culture starts with better conversations [Internet]. Greensboro: CCL; 2025. Available from: https://www.ccl.org.

25. Edmondson AC. The fearless organization: creating psychological safety in the workplace for learning, innovation, and growth. 1st ed. Hoboken: Wiley; 2018.

26. Luria S, Kaufman JC. The dynamic force before intrinsic motivation: exploring creative needs. In: Karwowski M, Kaufman JC, editors. The creative self: effect of beliefs, self-efficacy, mindset, and identity. Amsterdam: Academic Press; 2017.

27. Maslow A. Towards a psychology of being. 2nd ed. New York: Van Nostrand Reinhold; 1968.

28. Wilson C, Munn-Giddings C, Bungay H, Dadswell A. Arts, cultural and creative engagement during COVID-19: enhancing the mental wellbeing and social connectedness of university staff and students. Nord J Arts Cult Health. 2022;4(1):1–13. https://doi.org/10.18261/njach.4.1.2.

29. Beghetto RA. Creative learning: a fresh look. J Cogn Educ Psychol. 2016;25:6–23.

30. Tanggaard L, Glăveanu V. Creativity, identity, and representation: towards a socio-cultural theory of creative identity. New Ideas Psychol. 2014;34:12–21.

31. West M, Coia D. Caring for doctors, caring for patients: how to transform UK healthcare environments to support doctors and medical students to care for patients. London: General Medical Council; 2019. Available from: https://www.gmc-uk.org.

32. West M, Bailey S, Williams E. The courage of compassion: supporting nurses and midwives to deliver high-quality care. London: The King's Fund; 2020. Available from: https://www.kingsfund.org.uk/publications/courage-compassion-supporting-nurses-midwives.

33. Simonton DK. Domain-general creativity: on producing original, useful, and surprising combinations. In: Kaufman JC, Glăveanu VP, Baer J, editors. Cambridge handbook of creativity across different domains. New York: Cambridge University Press; 2017.

34. Maslow A. The farther reaches of human nature. New York: Viking; 1971.

35. Wallace DB, Gruber HE. The case study method and evolving systems approach for understanding unique creative people at work. In: Sternberg RJ, editor. Handbook of creativity. Cambridge: Cambridge University Press; 1999.

36. Anderson C, Cropley A. Correlates of originality. Aust J Psychiatry. 1966;18(1):218–27.

37. Wormington S. Better culture starts with compassionate leadership [Internet]. Greensboro: Center for Creative Leadership; 2024. Available from: https://www.ccl.org/articles/better-culture-starts-with-compassionate-leadership.

38. Royal College of Obstetricians and Gynaecologists. Improving workplace behaviours: workplace behaviour toolkit [Internet]. London: RCOG; 2021. Available from: https://www.rcog.org.uk/careers-and-training/workforce/improving-workplace-behaviours/workplace-behaviour-toolkit/.

39. Dubree M, Kapu A, Terrell M, Pichert JW, Cooper WO, Hickson GB. Promoting professionalism by sharing a cup of coffee. Am Nurse Today. 2017;12(5):18–9. Available from: https://www.americannursetoday.com.

40. Constructive Dialogue Institute. What is constructive dialogue? [Internet]. 2025. Available from: https://constructivedialogue.org.

41. Working Families. Working Families Index 2025: employer briefing [Internet]. London: Working Families; 2025. Available from: https://workingfamilies.org.uk.

42. NHS England. NHS health and wellbeing strategic overview [Internet]. London: NHS England; 2022. Available from: https://www.england.nhs.uk/publication/nhs-health-and-wellbeing-framework.

43. Ray TK, Pana-Cryan R. Work flexibility and work-related well-being. Int J Environ Res Public Health. 2021;18(6):3254. https://doi.org/10.3390/ijerph18063254.

44. Halpern DF. How time-flexible work policies can reduce stress, improve health, and save money. Stress Health. 2005;21(3):157–68. https://doi.org/10.1002/smi.1049.

45. Lacobucci G. Improving flexible working in the NHS. BMJ. 2023;380:618. https://doi.org/10.1136/bmj.p618.

46. Hutchings R, Lobont C, Fisher E, Palmer B. Future proof: the impact of parental and caring responsibilities on surgical careers. London: Nuffield Trust; 2023. Available from: https://www.nuffieldtrust.org.uk/research/future-proof-the-impact-of-parental-and-caring-responsibilities-on-surgical-careers.

47. Agyeman-Manu K, Ghebreyesus TA, Maait M, Rafila A, Tom L, Trindade Lima N, et al. Prioritising the health and care workforce shortage: protect, invest, together. Lancet Glob Health. 2023;11(8):e1162–4. Available from: https://www.thelancet.com/journals/langlo/article/PIIS2214-109X(23)00265-4/fulltext.

48. Radhakrishna S. Culture of blame in the National Health Service; consequences and solutions. Br J Anaesth. 2015;115(5):653–5. Available from: https://www.bjanaesthesia.org.

49. Horsfall S. Doctors who commit suicide while under GMC fitness to practise investigation: internal review. London: General Medical Council; 2014. Available from: https://www.gmc-uk.org.

50. NHS England. Patient safety incident response framework: oversight roles and responsibilities specification. Version 1. London: NHS England; 2022. Available from: https://www.england.nhs.uk/publication/patient-safety-incident-response-framework-supporting-guidance.

51. NHS England. 2024 National NHS staff survey results [Internet]. London: NHS England; 2025. Available from: https://www.nhsstaffsurveys.com/.

52. Independent Investigation into East Kent Maternity Services. Maternity and neonatal services in East Kent – the Report of the Independent Investigation. London:

GOV.UK; 2022. Available from: https://www.gov.uk/government/publications/maternity-and-neonatal-services-in-east-kent-reading-the-signals-report.

53. Independent Review of Maternity Services at Shrewsbury and Telford Hospital NHS Trust. Ockenden report: findings, conclusions and essential actions. London: GOV.UK; 2022. Available from: https://www.gov.uk/government/publications/final-report-of-the-ockenden-review.

54. The Mid Staffordshire NHS Foundation Trust Public Inquiry. Report of the mid Staffordshire NHS foundation trust public inquiry. London: GOV.UK; 2013. Available from: https://www.gov.uk/government/publications/report-of-the-mid-staffordshire-nhs-foundation-trust-public-inquiry.

55. Hanchett Hanson M, Amato A, Durani A, Hoyden J, Koe S, Sheagren E, Yang Y. Creativity and improvised educations: case studies for understanding impact and implications. London: Routledge; 2021.

56. Andina-Díaz E, et al. Lack of autonomy and professional recognition as major factors for burnout in midwives: a systematic mixed-method review. J Adv Nurs [Preprint]. 2024. https://doi.org/10.1111/jan.16279.

57. Simpson D, Hamilton S, McSherry R, McIntosh R. Measuring and assessing healthcare organisational culture in England's National Health Service: a snapshot of current tools and tool use. Healthcare (Basel). 2019;7(4):127. https://doi.org/10.3390/healthcare7040127. PMID: 31683839; PMCID: PMC6955975.

58. NHS England. NHS long term workforce plan [Internet]. London: NHS England; 2023. Available from: https://www.england.nhs.uk/publication/nhs-long-term-workforce-plan.

59. World Health Organization. Global strategy on human resources for health: workforce 2030 [Internet]. Geneva: WHO; 2016. Available from: https://www.who.int/publications/i/item/9789241511131.

5

Disconnected Policies and Tick Box Exercises: Understanding Politics, Process and Your Power

Introduction

Politics and policy in healthcare form a crucial part of the workplace culture. It includes the numerous micro-politics, policy-based operational processes and the policies themselves which can both exert power over and direct individual workers in their daily duties at work. Policies and politics also influence workplace behaviour and teamwork.

Power in this context can be summarised as an ability or capacity to achieve something, whether by influence or control, and political power can help us understand the workplace politics affecting individuals in their practice and decisions. This chapter explores the (often unspoken) powers, tensions and politics that either explicitly influence healthcare processes or implicitly create and shape powerful undercurrents in the workplace. The chapter aids you to reflect upon and understand your political position, power and influence and to identify how political factors direct your own thinking, decision-making and practice. Cases and examples from media and research prompt you to be politically curious, avoid ambivalent acceptance of politically based matters and develop courage to think and act in ways that enable and support positive culture in healthcare practice.

Healthcare organisations and the policies they implement, the way they invest in their workforce and how they manage workloads have a profound impact on patient safety, workplace culture and staff retention. It is important to critically assess whether all tasks required of healthcare professionals genuinely add value. Routine activities such as form-filling, ticking boxes and excessive documentation may not always contribute meaningfully to care delivery or staff wellbeing. In some cases, these tasks can become burdensome, detracting from time spent with patients and contributing to stress and burnout.

This raises an important question: Are all tasks truly beneficial, or are some simply fulfilling procedural requirements without improving outcomes? Creating space

L. Philp-von Woyna, *Unravelling Workplace Culture in Healthcare*,
https://doi.org/10.1007/978-3-032-11771-7_5

to evaluate the purpose and impact of such tasks is essential for streamlining workflows, supporting staff and ultimately enhancing the quality of care.

Information Chaos in Healthcare

A key challenge in healthcare relates to the volume of clinical documentation required; from recording patient history, repeating documentation in different software packages and completing endless checklists, the volume can be unmanageable. A new report from the National Academy of Medicine reveals that nurses and doctors spend approximately 50% of their working day documenting at the computer screen and not with the patient [1]. While the shift to electronic medical records (EMRs) was intended to streamline this process, some studies suggest the opposite has occurred. In fact, documentation burdens may have increased due to challenges in locating information, disrupted information flow and a lack of clinically focused organisation that supports effective decision-making [2].

In many ways, the introduction of EMRs has created a new set of problems that require smarter, more patient-centred technologies and systems that enhance information flow and support healthcare professionals in delivering timely, accurate care. Since documentation plays a critical role in clinical reasoning, EMRs must be designed to intelligently preserve and present key information to aid decision-making. Poor access to essential documentation can negatively impact patient outcomes, increase the risk of errors and medicolegal issues and disrupt continuity of care [2]. Furthermore, research suggests that inefficiencies in documentation and difficulties accessing relevant patient information may contribute to physician burnout [1].

The challenges associated with electronic medical records are an example of where there is a mandatory requirement to engage with a task (documentation via the organisations chosen electronic records system), regulatory penalties for non-compliance, but an overburdensome existing process that is arguably not fit for purpose and that can challenge effective clinical decision-making and time to care for patients. Existing healthcare policies and processes can, at times, present challenges that impact levels of stress within the workplace and subsequently workplace culture. More broadly politics, such as healthcare funding arrangements and responsiveness of broader national healthcare policy, can influence the workplace environment.

A recent study reported that healthcare workers are finding hospital shifts progressively more strenuous and stressful [3]. The number of people waiting in Accident and Emergency departments is increasing with long waiting times and delays [3]. Policy is partly to blame for underfunding spaces, resources and staffing to cope with increasing demand. and so it is important for healthcare professionals to understand policy, the ways to challenge it and how to participate in building policy that works.

Healthcare Policy Can Be Empowering or Disempowering

Policy often represents a series of power dynamics. Power dynamics in healthcare can be made known and analysed through the written workplace policies that can be both empowering and disempowering for differing staff groups and patients. Power refers to an ability or capacity to achieve something, whether by influence or control. Policies are written systems or texts that are symbols of cultural, moral and ethical values underpinned by political and professional agenda and law [4]. These values, political agendas and laws are sometimes in conflict with providing the *best* healthcare and in facilitating the wellbeing of staff.

Policy reflects power by placing emphasis on written texts to bring about change or practice [4]. In healthcare, policies are often written by those who hold a position of power with purpose to influence practice direction and implement ideas for solutions to a problem [5]. However, it is important to acknowledge that policies are not singular, one-way written processes that are unquestionably accepted by others and is essential to critically question the fit of policies for creating a positive healthcare culture. While policies detail a series of written ways to practice that often demand compliance, policy documents are received, interpreted and acted on in different ways by different groups. They do not always effectively establish norms or standards of practice but work dynamically in their influence on the practice of individuals. Policy texts can be both, or either, empowering or disempowering and this is temporal (related to the current context). For example, much pre-pandemic health policy has become both unrealistic and unachievable in the post-pandemic era without significant investment. Pre-pandemic health policy in the UK sets benchmark standards for acceptable patient waiting times for diagnostics. Pre-pandemic data shows that targets were largely met with most patients waiting less than 6 weeks for diagnostics and 6371 people waiting more than 13 weeks [6]. In 2024, the number of people waiting more than 13 weeks for diagnostics has risen to 118,212. This is problematic, not only in terms of the nation's health and the economic impact [6] but also in terms of impact on workplace culture.

Performance standards set in policy or processes which are unattainable for staff may contribute towards creating a narrative of a *failing service and failing culture* that can be disempowering for staff. In terms of applying pre-pandemic targets in a post-pandemic health service, this may account for the rising levels of healthcare worker 'burnout' and fatigue. Some studies have shown that post-pandemic, healthcare workers are stressed, overwhelmed and ready to leave their jobs [7]. However, rather than identifying as overwhelmed and burned out, some healthcare workers instead describe themselves as *demoralised* [8]. It is important to think about how policy might be contributing towards healthcare workplace culture that is as media portrays UK healthcare as *failing* and staff describe it as *demoralising*. Findings from my doctoral research with health students post-pandemic echoed these perspectives on workplace culture and provide insight into the impact of setting unachievable benchmarks.

One participant wrote,

[nobody] cares much…including the government. We've [student health professionals] been more affected [than most] by Coronavirus … [we] have lost…The decisions that are being made about our health education are important and will impact society and how well equipped it will be in the future. We are the future of healthcare. For things to be successful, you need people who feel supported by the government who are well equipped to then take and manage future generations. [9]

This statement suggests that policy (from the government) may improve health-care education and equip for the healthcare of the future. The participant proposes a solution that is focussed on ensuring health students feel supported and are well equipped to become *leaders* who are effective at managing the future demands of healthcare.

Many participating health students in the study were driven by a strong desire to make a meaningful impact [9]. They expressed a commitment to leading change and demonstrated a sense of civic responsibility in their professional roles. Their intentions extended beyond personal gain, focusing instead on supporting the wellbeing of both patients and colleagues, and prioritising broader societal health goals. These students also recognized the importance of policy that values their contributions and supports the future of healthcare. Consistent with existing literature, the study reinforces that without substantial investment in healthcare leadership education, equitable working conditions and fair compensation through national and local policy, retaining the healthcare workforce will remain a persistent challenge [10]. Box 5.1 invites you to reflect on how policy can influence these dynamics.

Box 5.1 Reflect on How Policy Influences Your Workplace Behaviour and Decisions

Think about a time when you have had a complex task or too many tasks and not enough time to complete them to a standard you were proud of.

1. How did you feel when you realised it was unachievable?
2. Think about the role certain policies, processes or standards may have contributed towards how you felt.
3. What changes to policies, processes or standards might have made you feel different?
4. What do you think needs to change?

Healthcare Policymaking and Creating

Policy can act as a type of power that supports change. Box 5.1 may have prompted you to think about what can be learned from aspects of policy that challenge you in clinical practice or where new policy may be needed. The critical study and analysis of health policy can reveal valuable insights into how existing policies and processes shape social and cultural behaviours within healthcare settings. This approach enables us to learn from current frameworks and identify areas for improvement. Furthermore, it helps to uncover the origins of policy development, highlighting the driving forces behind policy creation (the drivers) and the underlying rationale or justification for change (the warrant). Gillian Forrester, a professor of education policy, suggests policy is influenced by a range of factors that includes social, political, economic, technological, religious and cultural factors [11].

The origins of policymaking remain a subject of debate, with questions around whether it is primarily driven at the national level, shaped more locally or influenced by globalisation [12]. Some suggest the interests of 'supranational agents' or the spread of popular trends ('fads') can lead to global policy development or exert global influence, resulting in the transfer of policy ideas across borders [12]. This suggests that policy formation is dynamic and multifaceted, but various theories exist which attempt to explain how policies are shaped. For instance, pluralist theory proposes that policy is formed through equal input from a wide range of stakeholders, whereas elitist theory contends that a select, powerful few hold the most influence [13]. Additionally, the concept of co-optation highlights the role of regulatory or independent bodies in assisting governments, often through formal reports or procedures, in interpreting and implementing policy. This process can establish hierarchies and lend authority to certain policies and policy development [14].

Health policy is shaped through a variety of development pathways, often influenced by significant events or key reports. This means that anyone involved in delivering or receiving healthcare can play a role in guiding its direction and priorities. A recent example is Martha's Rule, which demonstrates how both individuals and organisations can impact the complex processes of policy formation and implementation. This case highlights the potential for *individual* experiences and advocacy to drive meaningful change within the healthcare system.

In 2021, Martha Mills, a 13-year-old girl, tragically died after developing sepsis in an English hospital. She had been admitted with a pancreatic injury after falling off her bike which initially was not thought to be life-threatening. She was transferred to a hospital in south London because it is one of three national centres for the care of children with pancreatic trauma. Despite this, Martha went on the develop sepsis which is treatable if acted upon early enough. Martha's parents reported their concerns that her health was deteriorating. However, their concerns were not heeded, and Martha's parents describe how nursing staff privately acknowledged Martha was at risk of dying, but doctors involved in her care only reassured them [15]. Martha's mother, Merope, considered whether doctors were trying not to worry her, but commented that doctors did not give any opportunity in agency to demand the correct treatment for their daughter. She commented on the power doctors held saying that a doctors control and overconfidence in themselves and their decision-making is absolutely fine if the system works perfectly, but the system is far from perfect [15].

In 2023, a UK coroner ruled that Martha would probably have survived had she been treated in a timely way and moved to intensive care earlier. Martha's case led to the Secretary of State for Health and Social Care and NHS England (NHSe) to commit to implementing *Martha's Rule. Martha's Rule* aims to ensure that the concerns of patients and their families are listened to and responded to. It sets out a series of actions that include improved access for patients and their families to raise concerns and be heard, placing emphasis on the concerns of patients and their families and improving access for all staff to seek a rapid review from critical care teams [16]. *Martha's Rule* informs national policy that is currently being introduced across the UK's health service from 2025.

Martha's mother, Merope, told a BBC reporter that instigating the process of seeking a second opinion should not be a problem for families and should not involve confrontation. Martha's Rule formalises the idea of asking for a second opinion when patients or their families do not feel as though they are being heard and provides an example of how policy can emerge from one individual and circumstance, even when there is a difference in *power*.

This case offers a valuable opportunity for reflection, as it demonstrates how learning from specific incidents or circumstances can inform and drive national health policy. While policy is often shaped by political values and motivations at various levels, feedback and action from individuals remains essential for meaningful improvement. As a healthcare worker, you play a crucial role in both motivating and mediating policy development. Like Martha's mother, individual voices can be highly influential in prompting policy change.

Box 5.2 encourages you to explore the details of Martha's case further and consider how individual agency can serve as a powerful force in shaping local and national healthcare policy.

Box 5.2 Reflecting on Martha's Rule and Individual Influence on Health Policy Development
1. Think about how the different people (below) were crucial to, and acted as, agents in the formation and ongoing implementation of Martha's Rule:
   - Martha's mother, Merope
   - The nurses caring for Martha
   - Media reporters
   - Secretary of State for Health and Social Care
   - NHS England
2. How could you take individual action towards policy development?

Understanding the Power of Politics and Policy in Healthcare

One prominent finding from my doctoral research centred around how politics and policy influenced the behaviour of individual healthcare students feeding into the broader learning culture [9]. Participants who shared ideas described aspects of external systems or powers as the factors which shaped and developed their thinking and ideas. Ideas were often politically mediated (shaped by politics whether that be local micropolitics or wider policy) and they were politically motivated. One participant shared an idea about how to address racism in maternity care, a subject of current political and social relevance [17]. One participant stated,

> I shared my idea for a plan which will focus on educating midwives on ethnicities, religions, and cultures to promote the understanding for when caring for women from ethnic minorities, the aim being to improve their experiences and tackle systemic racism…The programme will be a compulsory task that midwives need to carry out along with their mandatory training…. they should be recognising diversity and promoting individual choices. [9]

In the study, several similar examples illustrated associations between local politics, at university, among peers and in healthcare, national politics and sharing ideas that supported political views [9]. Solutions shared reflected existing local policy-based solutions and the broader political discourse because ideas promoted and sustained the established (normal or usual) way to deal with issues.

For example, in the case discussed, the student believed that making education about racism a compulsory task was the most effective way to address the issue, drawing from her own experience of mandatory training in maternity care. In some respects, compulsory tasks can be beneficial, as they signal a formal commitment to tackling a problem and demonstrate how policy (such as mandatory training) can support education and influence attitudes, behaviours and practices. However, relying solely on mandatory approaches may oversimplify complex issues, potentially limiting the development of more nuanced and diverse solutions. Reducing a multi-faceted problem to a single compulsory intervention risks overlooking the broader systemic and cultural changes that may be needed.

In my doctoral research, participants demonstrated contrasting approaches to problem-solving that reflected either collectivist or individualist orientations [9]. Those with collectivist views tended to prioritise societal benefit and favoured rule-based solutions that promoted compliance and consequences for non-adherence. These perspectives often aligned with conservative political beliefs and a preference for maintaining established systems. In contrast, participants with individualist views focused on personal autonomy, even when such approaches might not serve the broader collective. These differing orientations influenced not only their political leanings but also the way they generated and developed ideas, revealing distinct behavioural patterns tied to their underlying values and beliefs.

Some participants in the study used language such as 'tackle', 'compulsory task', 'mandatory' and 'should be', reflecting a preference for rule-based solutions to healthcare challenges. While these approaches aim to address problems decisively, they can also reinforce rigid, normalised responses that limit alternative thinking. Anderson and Cropley describe this phenomenon as 'cultural stops', behaviours that suppress diverse perspectives in favour of maintaining a singular viewpoint [18]. When policy solutions are framed in ways that demand strict compliance, they may become intolerant of other approaches, making noncompliance socially or professionally unacceptable. Although there may be consensus on the need to address a problem, it is important that solutions remain open to diverse and potentially more effective alternatives. This dynamic is particularly relevant in healthcare, where mandatory approaches are often modelled by those in authority. In the example cited, a student's views were shaped by recent exposure to compulsory university training on systemic racism, illustrating how institutional practices can influence individual perspectives on problem-solving.

In contrast to mandatory, rule-based approaches to problem-solving, some participants in my doctoral study expressed more liberal and open-minded perspectives. These individuals were more tolerant of differing views and preferred exploring complex, inclusive solutions that considered the holistic needs of others. While mandatory policies can offer clear advantages, such as consistency and accountability, they may also limit innovation and suppress alternative viewpoints. Participants with liberal views tended to favour collaborative problem-solving and were more willing to engage with diverse perspectives [9].

Box 5.3 encourages reflection on how you personally approach policy-based solutions, helping you critically evaluate both the strengths and limitations of mandatory versus flexible approaches.

Box 5.3 Analysing Your Own Health Policy-Based Ideas

1. Think about a problem that you would like to see addressed through a new healthcare-related policy.
2. What is the main purpose of the policy? What would you like to achieve? And how could this be addressed through the policy?
3. Reflect on the potential strengths and limitations of your policy idea based on each point detailed in the table below. This will enable you to identify the potential strengths and weaknesses of your policy-based idea.

	Potential strengths	Potential limitations
Mandatory actions are part of your idea You might have included a mandatory checklist that forms part of your policy idea	Mandatory compliance is more likely to achieve a controlled measurable outcome. This can be advantageous in circumstances where a measurable difference is required to be evidenced	The mandatory solution or checklist might not actually address the problem you intend to address. Think about whether it truly addresses the problem A mandatory solution demands compliance which can reduce individual autonomy and *models* regulated ways to deal with problems. It models that mandatory compliance is an appropriate way to meet the aim/ solve the problem. Think about whether you want to reduce individual autonomy and reduce diversity of approaches to solving the problem with the introduction of *one mandatory way/one checklist* to solve the problem

	Potential strengths	Potential limitations
Rewards and sanctions are part of your policy-based idea	Rewards and sanctions can improve compliance At times, rewards and sanctions can improve motivation for compliance	Drives solutions in one direction which may not address the problem Excessive reliance on external motivators such as rewards and sanctions can undermine individual intrinsic motivation, leading to decreased engagement and satisfaction Overreliance on rewards or sanctions may reduce engagement in idea-sharing Rewards and sanctions may be perceived as coercive and if applied unfairly or inconsistently can foster distrust and resentment Behaviours that model 'reward or sanction' promote these behaviours in other areas of policy development
Your policy-based idea is broad, open and inclusive and involves individuals making a judgement or contribution within boundaries that are somewhat flexible	Improves individual and group autonomy to meet the policy requirements Promotes and motivates idea-sharing for meeting the policy Promotes flexibility and openness in searching for solutions to other problems Improves individualised approaches to problems, that are context specific and/or individualised to patients	There is less control over measurable outcomes Intended outcomes might not be achieved Policy discourse may become a problem because it becomes a product of language that is shaped by social interaction with the policy Power dynamics can be become an issue in policy because certain voices and perspectives over its implementation and outcomes can take the lead This approach is more likely to be influenced by local values and interpretations in-context shaping the direction of policy informed action

4. By reflecting on the main points in the table, how could you strengthen your policy-based idea and share it in your workplace?

In completing Box 5.3, you will have gained understanding about how policy formation can contribute towards influencing the workplace climate/culture. Policies and policy-based ideas that involve more control (power) leave less room for development of new ideas or solutions to emerge. While approaching problems in a way that demands compliance with policy-based action may include sanctions and rewards, it introduces the risk of being disconnected from individuals and treating problems as objective issues that require management rather than problems that involve how people work together, as individuals part of a wider systems and team. In contrast, where policy introduces more scope for individual ideas to emerge, there is less control (power) in achieving a measurable outcome. Approaching problems in a way that introduces policy that exerts less control may mean there is less certainty about whether the problem will be addressed, and it may also introduce discourse with unintended consequences.

Power dynamics in policy formation significantly influence what policies can be achieved, particularly when those crafting policy holds dominant positions. When policy is shaped primarily by individuals in power, it often leads to reduced tolerance for alternative viewpoints and can instil fear in those wishing to propose different approaches [19]. This disconnect between policymakers and frontline healthcare workers can result in rigid, less inclusive policies that fail to reflect the realities of everyday practice. Fear of social rejection, rooted in concerns about how ideas will be received can suppress innovation and limit the diversity of ideas. Research across decades has shown that social acceptance plays a critical role in shaping whether individuals feel safe to share their perspectives, especially in cultures or workplaces with strong norms [18–20]. Addressing these power imbalances and fostering environments that welcome diverse input is essential for developing robust, responsive healthcare policies.

Findings from my doctoral research as well as existing literature recognises that both intrinsic and extrinsic factors work together to influence behaviour, contributions to problem-solving and policy in healthcare [9, 21]. While policy is an external factor that influences how individuals act and make decisions, it also influences how individuals intrinsically feel and respond to problems in the future [9, 21]. As outlined in Box 5.3, policy has the potential to increase or decrease job satisfaction, increase or decrease social and group-based action and alter the way individuals feel about work, including their motivation at work and whether they develop feelings of distrust.

The tension between intrinsic motivation and external demands plays a significant role in shaping how healthcare professionals share ideas, take action and contribute to innovation and policy [21]. Personal values, desires and traits, rooted in a sense of purpose, can sometimes conflict with systemic expectations, particularly when policy dictates rigid practices that limit autonomy [20]. For example, a health worker may wish to provide more personalised care but is constrained by policies that prioritise resource, efficiency and documentation. These tensions can lead to reduced job satisfaction, fear of noncompliance and reluctance to share ideas for improvement. Addressing these challenges begins with recognising one's own position and influence and understanding the wider political, cultural and structural dynamics within and outside the healthcare system locally, nationally and internationally.

Box 5.4 invites reflection on how policy is shaped in local and wider contexts and how it impacts different groups, encouraging a more critical and inclusive approach to policy development.

> **Box 5.4 Policy Formation and Development in the Local and Wider Context**
>
> Health is unequally distributed society, locally and globally with some individuals or groups having more of it than others. Political interventions can alter the health of groups and individuals and policy on both the local and global level matter for this reason. For instance, policymakers may be mandated to devise or revise policy by *supranational* institutions, such as in the case of European regulations like the General Data Protection Regulation (GDPR). This might directly influence how care can be organised locally [22]. Local policy is connected and influenced by global policy meaning understanding of both is crucial in the development of new policy or revision of existing policy. Policy development in the local context typically happens through one or more of the following ways:
>
> 1. Through coercive top-down implementation where policymakers simply mandate a particular course of action
> 2. Through bottom-up implementation where policymakers create the right circumstances to encourage professionals to voluntarily work together to develop policy
> 3. Through a consultative approach, where policymakers consult with particular interest groups or expert panels make decisions
> 4. Through wider mandated action where policymakers devise or revise policy according to supranational institutions
>   (i) In what ways can you contribute towards local, national or international health policy development?
>   (ii) How can you empower others (particularly those who hold positions with less power than you) to also contribute towards policy development?

To bring policy-based ideas and challenge the ways in which problems are addressed through policy and other means, understanding your own power in influencing ideas becomes necessary [23]. Individual healthcare professionals operate within a broader community where their ability to share creative ideas is shaped by their position and the surrounding dynamics of power, meaning and value. Contributing innovative solutions often involves navigating uncertainty and risk and requires a strong sense of autonomy and self-belief [24, 25]. The decision to share an idea is often influenced by an individual's sense of autonomy [26], as well as their ability to judge the right time, place and context for doing so [27]. In healthcare, understanding the workplace culture and broader system dynamics can help individuals recognise the power structures that shape their environment and identify opportunities to challenge or disrupt them through idea-sharing [20, 24]. Enhancing students awareness of political culture, debate and policy discourse may empower more creative contributions by helping them understand their own position and influence within these systems and policy.

Strategies that are relatively simple can disrupt local social tensions, group dynamics, and access to tools that support negotiation in practice and policy. For example, in healthcare, tools like the 'teach or treat?' strategy [28] can help disrupt hierarchical norms by encouraging open discussion about clinical decisions. This simple question fosters mutual understanding and learning across roles, by having conversations about why treatment is or is not recommended, though it requires courage to raise potentially challenging issues. Enabling and encouraging others to participate in problem-solving, and including diverse perspectives in policy development leads to more informed and effective solutions [9]. This was evidenced in my doctoral research, with examples of how encouraging, empowering and facilitating the involvement of others in problem-solving led to better informed and more robust solutions beneficial in policy development. One participant wrote,

> [We]…created a mind map of issues… about how to create something to turn this [the problem] around…Together we recognised the issues…and discussed ideas on how to change [it]… It was a team effort, and I really enjoy discussing these topics in this way with others. It is so insightful to hear so many different views on the same topic. [9]

Their contributions reflected *collective creativity*, where ideas were shaped not solely by the individual but through the opportunities and influences present in their social and contextual environment. These findings highlight that embracing diverse viewpoints and the complexity of differing personalities and perspectives can enrich and enhance outcomes, including policy ideas and development.

Thinking Critically About How Policy and Tick-Box Agendas Influence Workplace Culture

Some view implementation of policy as separate from the policymaking process, whereas others view it as part of the whole dynamic process [29]. While some suggest the implementation of policy includes the process of interactions that starts with setting goals and results in action to achieve the goals [30], others view it as a more dynamic process [31]. This is because policy is *interpreted and translated* into actionable points in the context of the institution and as restrained by discourses [31]. Therefore, critically considering the context of policymaking aids understanding about the influencing factors and discourses in the creation, interpretation, enactment *and* implementation of policy. There are numerous theories and frameworks available to critically examine existing written policies. Engaging in this kind of analysis is valuable not only for understanding how policy contributes to governance but also for exploring its real-world implications. It allows for deeper insight into how policy decisions affect practice and can guide future policy development. Additionally, critical analysis supports informed debate around the issues addressed in policy, helping to refine and improve its relevance and effectiveness.

An essential aspect to consider in the analysis of existing written policy is policy drivers. This involves asking questions about why a policy was formed. Analysis of policy drivers can include consideration of deficits (a problem created by a lack of) or excesses (a problem created by too much of) that led to policy formation [32]. Rational- purposive models of policy analysis suggest that policy formation will follow a clearly defined path, which starts with carefully considered intentions of those in formal positions of power, in response to problems [29]. These models suggest policy is simply a response to the problem, where a vision for the solution is encapsulated in a formal policy document with intended goals. Rational models also suggest levers (instruments available to those in power) are used to ensure compliance or shape change through rewards or sanctions [33]. A major criticism of defining and viewing policy through the rational-purposive model is that it fails to capture the 'messiness' of policymaking and implementation [29]. Alternative models such as those based on *discourse theory* view policy as more complex or organic. Through this perspective, policymaking and implementation is almost merged, where it is viewed as a whole dynamic process [29]. Dynamic views of policymaking and implementation suggest policy is an ongoing process, which is as much about the conflict, interpretation and complexity of implementation, as about the written text presented in a physical policy document. When thinking critically about policy, these factors can be considered to identify where and how policymaking and its implementation can be improved.

In addition, considering whether policy is written rationally by leaders in response to a problem, critique of the drivers, the levers and the dynamic emerging in policymaking and implementation can uncover policy discourse. Some describe the ongoing state of policy as 'policy discourse'; the idea that sociopolitical values inform dominant discourses that establish the strategic direction of policy and translate policy into the written text and subsequent practice. Policy discourse as a central concept of the policy process is a common theme in literature, and various aspects are thought to influence the dynamic process of policymaking and implementation, through discourse. From a theory discourse perspective, the policy is not viewed as merely a product, but consideration policies are texts being shaped by discourse and relations of power [34]. Each potential area of policy discourse can be considered in the critical analysis of policy and may be understood through analysing the language of policy that can reveal how competing powers have influenced it.

The Language of Policy Matters

Analysing the *language* used in or around policy is a valuable way to uncover the types of discourse that have shaped and influenced its development. The specific choice of words can reveal underlying power dynamics within both policy texts and the broader literature that supports them. In health, there are obvious and less obvious examples of where choice of *language* uncovers issues of a social, political and cultural nature. One such example relates to a recent publication in the esteemed British Medical Journal, The Lancet [35].

In September 2021, The Lancet featured a cover page with the statement 'Historically, the anatomy and physiology of bodies with vaginas have been neglected'. The cover attracted mixed opinions on social media with most condemning the language chosen. At the root of the social media debate was a deeper, culturally mediated and problematic truth, and the chosen language was a manifestation and surfacing of this social truth. In the context of healthcare, several studies highlight that *norms* surrounding usual clinical language can sustain inequalities, impact care and perpetually favour certain staff and patient groups, most often men and White, middle class, heterosexual people. The Lancet had (perhaps unintentionally) joined a narrative that *dehumanised* women and girls through language choice. Calling women, girls and transgender men '*bodies with vaginas*' reinforced an existing gender and sex inequality.

Following the incident, The Lancet apologised, claiming it was not intended to marginalise women and that they strive for maximum inclusivity of all people [36]. They highlighted that the intention was to emphasise that transgender health is an important and often neglected dimension of modern healthcare. Many agree with the response statement, but entirely erasing sex and gender in favour of the term *bodies* provides an interesting example of when language choice might contribute towards culture-based, social and political issues.

Conceptualisation of language theory suggests that the language we choose reflects the truth about the attitudes we hold and the discourses we subscribe to. We may also imitate language heard that unintentionally becomes part of a wider narrative contributing towards and perpetuating inequality. If *bodies with vaginas* became an accepted language norm, it has social and cultural consequences. Language influences how we think and then subsequently how we act. In modern healthcare, there is a recent increase in discussions surrounding language, what the 'right' word to use is and what the 'wrong' word is. However, attempts at finding the perfect answer and/or breaking down problematic normative use of language in healthcare often provoke feelings of uncertainty for individuals.

Language is a connection to social relations as constructed by society [37]. Through language, knowledge and understanding is shaped and so what language is chosen matters in policy and literature [34]. Policies use language as power and as a tool to influence others. A policy may use naturalisation which conditions society to accept language, ideas and practices, which might or might not be in their best interests [37]. The language used is often presented as 'common sense' making it difficult for others to challenge. Analysing language in health policy and, in particular, the narrative it creates for different groups and the inequalities it may contribute towards is an important part of policy analysis because language is used to construct convincing realities, which presuppose or imply a situation, which is not necessarily true [34].

Analysing issue rhetoric is a further aspect of policy, which refers to how language frames problems, often narrowing them down to specific, seemingly technical concerns, such as deteriorating hospital infrastructure or unsafe equipment [32]. Evaluating whether rhetoric is grounded in evidence and philosophical reasoning or shaped by political agendas can help determine the *authenticity and relevance* of the problem being addressed in a policy. This is sometimes referred to as 'legitimisation', the process by which policies are justified by aligning with dominant norms and values [34]. One form of legitimisation is authorisation, where policies gain legitimacy through authoritative means, such as being embedded in law, making them difficult to challenge [34]. The reasoning and factors of legitimisation are useful in understanding how language and agenda influences healthcare policy and practice and how it shapes priorities and decision-making.

The language used in healthcare, both social and clinical, serves as a lens through which cultural and societal realities within practice can be examined. Linguistic theory supports the idea that the selection of specific terms and expressions can reveal underlying social truths, offering valuable insights that can inform and enhance healthcare policy development.

Micro-politics in Healthcare

In my doctoral study, local culture and micro-politics influenced whether ideas to improve healthcare were shared and how those ideas developed and were supported [9]. Micro-politics is about the *everyday* politics in the local setting, rather than the broader politics discussed so far in this chapter that is often made known through health policy. Everyday micro-politics include how power dynamics play out in the local healthcare setting or ward environment through communication and conflict between individuals. Micro-politics is about how power is used in the workplace (by those in positions of power) such as shift leaders and/or those in higher hierarchical positions to control relationships with colleagues and team decisions. Micro-politics are *local* power-based factors that influence the local workplace culture. Examining and reflecting on micro-political factors can uncover entrenched, local culture-based issues.

Micro-politics that could be problematic include behaviours such as manipulation of others or overpowering others and restricting their autonomy. Behaviours like this might manifest in situations such as a shift leader assigning an unfair workload to a junior member of staff while favouring those in the team with more experience/power or overpowering a junior member of staff surrounding a decision they have made. These politics in the local workplace are a display (and sometimes misuse) of power by those with more power, and it may build and sustain problems in local workplace culture. In my doctoral study, cases demonstrated that the micro-political culture and broader politics (policy, political issues) both influenced healthcare worker motivation and willingness to share ideas for improvements [9]. In some cases, broad political focus, such as recent maternity safety investigations, influenced the ways in which individuals wanted to improve healthcare while the local micro-politics were important in facilitating whether individuals felt their ideas were valuable and could improve aspects of care [9].

Participants in my study shared ideas that included ways to address 'racial inequalities in maternity care', ideas that 'promoted culturally sensitive care', ideas that ensured 'more staff are trained correctly' and ideas that addressed the 'workforce struggling to find replacement staff to cover colleagues training needs' [9]. These ideas represent what was politically current (in the moment) as evidenced in national politics evident in midwifery reports, news and practice-related publications. The finding suggests that current issues in midwifery care, as featured in policy materials, midwifery reports and midwifery literature may highlight current problems that can act as a starting point for improvements and prompt creative thought about possible solutions. It suggests that current challenges can act as a form of motivation for creative ideas and action. However, cases also demonstrated that creative contributions may be constrained locally by conflicts with professional autonomy and the distribution of power within healthcare systems.

Although students participating in the study had ideas to address broad issues in maternity care, the local context often limited the sharing of ideas because there was a lack of opportunity to share ideas or colleagues in the local context used their power to shut down ideas [9]. Both *issues of power* and *ability to act autonomously* were micro-political issues that influenced ideas. For example, one participant described an idea about extending the length of postnatal maternity care support offered by midwives. Local healthcare policy constrained the idea because local protocol stated that women should be discharged at 10–14 days after birth, and this was in direct conflict with the idea presented by the student. Broader policy and funding arrangements also constrained the idea. Interestingly, while there was agreeance and support at the local and social level, senior colleagues advised the student that her idea would never be supported more widely because of resource constraints. Locally, the way postnatal care was provided up to 10–14 days was fully accepted as the norm by experienced midwives, they did not support or see opportunity for this aspect of care to change and therefore they played a role in shutting down the idea and sustaining norms around postnatal care provision.

The case provides an example about how the *local micro-politics* (how senior midwives use their power to influence others) can influence improvements in practice and idea-sharing, but also how broader policy affects improvement efforts. How senior colleagues respond to new ideas, problem solving, questioning and the challenging of norms by more junior staff was extremely influential in enabling and building a culture of learning and improvement. This aligns with wider literature that has examined why healthcare improvements fail or culture-based problems exist and persist in healthcare. Both my research and wider literature suggests that experienced staff (working locally) significantly influence the thought processes, idea-sharing and what healthcare improvements happen in those contexts [9, 18, 23, 25]. This supports that further research and/or interventions for healthcare improvements focussed on experienced professionals learning to be open, recognise the potential to learn from junior others and use their power to invest and collaborate with junior staff in making improvements happen may be beneficial.

Recent health-based investigation reports support this view, such as the Ockenden Report [38] and the Kirkup report [39] that investigated poor outcomes in maternity services at Shrewsbury and Telford NHS and East Kent NHS trusts. The Kirkup report found that seniors play a significant role in the practice and culture of practicing junior staff [39]; it states,

> What we saw and heard was that it was when clinicians were exposed to the behaviour of senior colleagues that their standards began to slip…If those role models themselves display poor behaviours, the potential is there for a negative cycle of declining standards. [39]

The Ockenden Report [38] discussed the barriers to improving care as including a lack of responsiveness from senior staff that led to the avoidable deaths and harm of mothers and babies. It states,

> [there were]…delays in escalation and failure to work collaboratively across disciplines, [that] resulted in the many poor outcomes… Some of the causes of these delays were due to the culture among the trust's workforce…there was a lack of action from senior clinicians following escalation. [38]

Role Modelling to Support a Learning Culture

In my doctoral research, local role modelling by experienced healthcare professionals was found to be influential across all cases and ideas shared in the study [9]. This included modelling in response to political matters or modelling about how individuals should act/behave within the local culture (how teams or groups work together including their shared values, attitudes and goals). Cases illustrated that the modelled and established culture of groups can either enable or constrain idea-sharing because individuals prefer their ideas to *fit in* with the established values, attitudes and goals of the group [9]. Cases illustrated that individuals *join the local in-group* culture (norms in group operation, politics and power) that reflect tensions about what kind of ideas, attitudes and behaviours are and are not acceptable to bring and from who. This matters in healthcare because it may help to explain why new ideas and creative contributions that intend to challenge poor healthcare practice might be squashed in established group cultures, as influenced by the unique micro-politics that exist in those groups. The micro-political environment can mean that some individuals use power to undermine others' autonomy limiting their confidence to share ideas and act on ideas to improve care. This might lead to more junior healthcare workers accepting local norms (ways of working) even when existing norms might be problematic. It becomes easier for junior staff to accept the norms and learn to behave in the same way because efforts to challenge norms are squashed by those in positions of power [18].

A lack of autonomy for individuals to express opinions and ideas and act upon them within the scope of their role not only constrains ideas but may also constrain future creative efforts, innovation, effective teamworking, workforce resilience and sense of wellbeing [20]. In my doctoral research, senior healthcare workers were more influential in both the development of ideas, what actions come from ideas and the confidence that individuals felt to share ideas. The conversations between senior and junior healthcare staff were found to be enabling for professional development, wellbeing and facilitating improvement ideas.

Box 5.5 encourages reflection on workplace micro-politics and its relationship to power-based and principle-based approaches to care, as well as broader workplace culture. This task draws on the Nimrod Review, an independent aviation report investigating the loss of the RAF Nimrod MR2 aircraft XV230 in Afghanistan in 2006 [40]. The review highlights how systemic cultural and organisational factors contributed to the incident. By examining these findings, healthcare professionals can identify parallels within healthcare settings, particularly regarding how workplace culture, communication and leadership influence safety and decision-making. Some of the Nimrod Review's recommendations offer valuable insights for shaping healthcare policy, especially in fostering cultures of accountability, transparency and continuous learning.

Box 5.5 Power-Based vs. Principle-Based Micro-politics in the Workplace

The Nimrod Review [40] strongly advocates for principle-based practice, offering a compelling contrast to rule-bound or compliance-driven approaches. Its findings highlight how organisational culture and decision-making frameworks contributed to a major incident, underscoring the importance of values-led leadership and accountability. Translating these principles into the healthcare context provides an opportunity to reflect on how policy is shaped, not just by regulations but by the underlying culture and ethical foundations of care. This cross-sector insight demonstrates the value of learning from other industries, reinforcing the need for healthcare policy formation and implementation to be informed by broad, interdisciplinary perspectives that prioritise safety, transparency and professional integrity.

1. The Nimrod Review advocates for *principles* over *procedures*. By embedding principle-based practice, such as accountability (being responsible for our own actions and decisions), transparency (being straightforward with others) and integrity (honest, ethical decision-making), safety and workplace culture can be improved [40].

   Where *principles* become more important than following *procedure,* the focus moves away from compliance towards genuinely understanding and mitigating risks as a team. For example, if a shift leader assigns higher workload to junior staff (an example of where power/micro-politics might manifest), principle-focussed team working might discuss the safety of this decision with the shift leader. Principle-focussed practice would hold *the team* accountable for decisions, not just the leader.

   Can you think of a similar workplace tension where principle-focussed practice may help to challenge workplace micro-politics?

2. **Empowerment and Responsibility in Principle-Based Practice**. The Nimrod Review [40] highlights that even when procedures are followed, risks exist and so everyone has a responsibility to raise when a risk is identified.

   In healthcare, this could mean following processes such as following a hospital policy or escalating a concern about a patient in the right way means that risks and safety issues will still be present. Therefore, everyone should feel empowered and responsible to speak up about potential risks.

Can you think of a time when you or a colleague followed a policy or process of escalation that did not entirely mitigate a risk?

3. **Ethical Leadership and Systemic Thinking in Principle-Based Practice**. The Nimrod Review [40] highlights the importance of role-modelled behaviour from leaders and demands that safety should be treated as a *moral obligation*. This principle should apply to all levels of a system and should focus on long-term *safety integrity* across all levels of an organisation rather than compliance across all levels.

   An expected principle of safety as a *moral obligation* for leaders in healthcare has the potential to refocus learning from incidents on *long-term safety integrity*, rather than blame and compliance. In healthcare, a blame culture and one that measures and values compliance over ethical and moral obligations and safety integrity can present challenges. For example, if concerns are raised about the care provided by a colleague, focus might be given to whether the person complied with policy and process rather than focus given to the principles of care they provided, the *safety integrity* of it, the leaders influencing their decisions and role-modelled behaviours they have experienced. The latter can provide better insight into *how* the *culture within the system* has enabled the error or practice to occur.

4. **Continuous Learning and Adaptation**. *Principle-based practice* supports a learning culture where feedback and incident analysis lead to meaningful change. It discourages complacency and promotes critical thinking about safety risks. *Principle-based practice* analyses the principles that individuals are working by, rather than their compliance with rules, policies or processes. It can aid understanding about what principles the organisation is working by and in doing so provides insight into how culture-based factors may be contributing towards incidents.

   Think of a workplace error or failure and reflect on the *principles* the individuals and teams involved in the error were working in accordance with. What can this tell you about the team culture-based factors that may have contributed towards the incident?

A *power-based* micro-political environment will measure and value compliance with hierarchy and by policy compliance. In contrast, a *principle-based* micro-political environment will examine the culture-based principles that are influencing workplace behaviour.

5. What power-based and principle-based practice have you observed in your workplace? How do you think principle-based practice could be improved?

Politics and Healthcare Education

In my doctoral study, the power of policy, politically commissioned health reports and political modelling in higher education was found to influence ideas formed and shared by student health professionals [9]. Like in the healthcare practice context, the local political culture in higher education enabled or constrained idea-sharing between students and in healthcare by students. Specifically, student midwives were motivated by current political issues but also vulnerable to sharing ideas that aligned with political discourse and the beliefs and values of their teachers [9]. Creative ideas often aligned with local dominant political discourse but, at times, aimed to challenge it.

Evidence suggests that individuals can successfully practice creatively sharing ideas, if and only if there are no substantial obstacles in the society (social context) preventing them [41]. In my doctoral research, ideas for healthcare improvement were found in part, at least, to be censored by common policy-based or political-based themes of the time and *place* [9]. It means that higher education (as a political place) plays a critical role in shaping ideas and facilitating a culture of learning and improvement.

A recent systematic review of creative pedagogical (teaching) practices summarised that 22 studies support opportunity to explore and generate ideas through openness in the classroom that can aid wider idea-sharing [42]. This finding is supported by others, who agree that teaching practices which enable student freedom of expression about ideas are beneficial to enable creativity and to generate creative solutions [43, 44]. In education, approaches that provide this freedom and openness, but are balanced with structure to classroom tasks, offer the most benefit in facilitating creative thought and action [42–44]. Cases in my doctoral study illustrate that student health professionals were open towards finding creative new ways of working and exploring creative solutions to problems with peers and teachers, but experienced censorship and shutting down of those ideas in clinical practice [9]. Extracts from cases shared illustrate how politics and micro-politics as facilitated by senior midwives, peers and local hospital policy played a role in shutting down some ideas, while upholding other ideas [9].

The political and micro-political landscape in clinical practice might limit idea-sharing opportunities. This matters because idea-sharing is essential as a prerequisite for improvement and innovation and is associated with individual wellbeing. A systematic review undertaken in 2024 examined why midwives experience burnout and might choose to leave the profession [45]. They found that burnout was associated with reduced individual self-confidence, empowerment and autonomy, but also with high rates of staff turnover and a reduction in the quality and safety of care provided by midwives. Burnout is associated with low personal fulfilment [46], whereas creative expression, the sharing of ideas and learning along with autonomy are associated with self-actualisation and high levels of fulfilment and purpose.

Providing opportunities for student health professionals and health professionals thereafter with spaces to think of and share creative solutions to current healthcare challenges may be beneficial not only for improving healthcare but also improving the retention of health professionals after they join the workforce. Fostering of creative cognitive skills among health professionals includes promoting the creative thinking (imagination) required in forming ideas with curiosity, reasoning and courage to take risks in sharing ideas [47]. Students, in particular, are well placed to bring fresh ideas, critical thoughts and problem-solving ideas to provide solutions [47] because theory suggests that students are positioned in a unique space of development where professional identity is forming but has not yet reached a point where it upholds the established culture. Participation with behaviours of senior colleagues and learning from them shapes the local culture [25], and this understanding can inform opportunities to disrupt local culture-based problems.

Summary

My doctoral research illustrated how student health professionals are motivated to act and address problems that are highlighted as issues in national and wider policy and/or in politically commissioned reports. In this way, the political and policy context influences the efforts in creative idea-sharing and changing practice. However, findings also suggest that factors in the local micro-political environment in clinical practice and higher education influence idea-sharing and action as well as individual wellbeing and achievement. This chapter has discussed the ways in which individuals can influence and participate in the formation and enactment of local and wider policy. Power, local micro-political influences and wider political issues and policies play a role in building workplace culture. It is therefore an essential aspect to examine and change when aiming to influence and change workplace culture.

References

1. Honavar SG. Electronic medical records – the good, the bad and the ugly. Indian J Ophthalmol. 2020;68(3):417–8. https://doi.org/10.4103/ijo.IJO_278_20. PMID: 32056991; PMCID: PMC7043175

2. Steinkamp J, Sharma A, Bala W, Kantrowitz JJ. A fully collaborative, noteless electronic medical record designed to minimize information chaos: software design and feasibility study. JMIR Form Res. 2021;5(11):e23789. https://doi.org/10.2196/23789. PMID: 34751651; PMCID: PMC8663541

3. NHS England. Monthly operational statistics – January 2025 [Internet]. London: NHS England; 2025. Available from: https://www.england.nhs.uk/statistics/

4. Stilz A. Decolonisation and self determination. Soc Philos Policy. 2015;32(1):1–24.

5. Topp SM, Schaaf M, Sriram V, Scott K, Dalglish SL, Nelson EM, et al. Power analysis in health policy and systems research: a guide to research conceptualisation. BMJ Glob Health. 2021;6(11):e007268. https://doi.org/10.1136/bmjgh-2021-007268. PMID: 34740915; PMCID: PMC8573637

6. NHS England. Diagnostic waiting times and activity data: November 2024 monthly report [Internet]. London: NHS England; 2025. Available from: https://www.england.nhs.uk/statistics/

7. Dunn P, Ewbank L, Alderwick H. Nine major challenges facing health and care in England. London: The Health Foundation; 2023. Available from: https://www.health.org.uk/reports-and-analysis/briefings/nine-major-challenges-facing-health-and-care-in-england

8. Hostetter M, Klein S. Responding to burnout and moral injury among clinicians [Internet]. New York: The Commonwealth Fund; 2023. Available from: https://doi.org/10.26099/k72x-t469

9. Philp-Von Woyna L. A multi-case study to understand the ways in which sociocultural factors influence everyday creative contributions in healthcare and higher education by student midwives [doctoral thesis]. Staffordshire: Staffordshire University; 2025. Available from: https://eprints.staffs.ac.uk/8884/

10. NHS England. NHS Long Term Workforce Plan [Internet]. London: NHS England; 2023. Available from: https://www.england.nhs.uk/publication/nhs-long-term-workforce-plan

11. Forrester G, Garratt D. Education policy unravelled. 2nd ed. London: Bloomsbury; 2016.

12. Ball S. The education debate. 2nd ed. Bristol: Policy Press; 2013.

13. Hewitt C. Pluralism in British policy-making: a reply to Morriss. Br J Polit Sci. 1976;6(3):351–6. Available from: http://www.jstor.org.libezproxy.open.ac.uk/stable/193655

14. Becher T, Kogan M. Process and structure in higher education. Milton Keynes: Open University Press; 1992.

15. Cursino M. Martha's rule: mother to press health secretary on patient rights [Internet]. London: BBC News; 2023. Available from: https://www.bbc.co.uk/news

16. NHS England. Implementation of first phase of Martha's Rule [Internet]. London: NHS England; 2024. Available from: https://www.england.nhs.uk/

17. HM Government. Inclusive Britain: government response to the Commission on Race and Ethnic Disparities [Internet]. London: HM Government; 2022. Available from: https://www.gov.uk/government/publications/inclusive-britain-government-response-to-the-commission-on-race-and-ethnic-disparities

18. Anderson C, Cropley A. Correlates of originality. Aust J Psychiatry. 1966;18(1):218–27.

19. Maslow A. The farther reaches of human nature. New York: Viking; 1971.

20. Runco M. Creativity: research, development, and practice. London: Elsevier Science; 2023.

21. Hanchett Hanson M, Amato A, Durani A, Hoyden J, Koe S, Sheagren E, Yang Y. Creativity and improvised educations: case studies for understanding impact and implications. London: Routledge; 2021.

22. Raus K, Mortier E, Eeckloo K. Challenges in turning a great idea into great health policy: the case of integrated care. BMC Health Serv Res. 2020;20(1):130. https://doi.org/10.1186/s12913-020-4950-z. PMID: 32085770; PMCID: PMC7035709

23. Hanchett HM. Author, self, monster: using Foucault to examine functions of creativity. J Theor Philos Psychol. 2013;33(1):18–31.

24. Beghetto RA. Creative learning: a fresh look. J Cogn Educ Psychol. 2016;25:6–23.

25. Lave J, Wenger E. Situated learning: legitimate peripheral participation. Cambridge: Cambridge University Press; 1991.

26. Rinne T, Daniel G, Fairweather J. The role of Hofstede's individualism in national-level creativity. Creat Res J. 2013;25(1):129–36.

27. Kaufman J, Beghetto RA. Where is the when of creativity? Specifying the temporal dimension of the Four Cs of creativity. Rev Gen Psychol. 2023;27(2):194–205.

28. Royal College of Obstetricians and Gynaecologists. Teach or treat [Internet]. London: RCOG. Available from: https://www.rcog.org.uk/about-us/quality-improvement-clinical-audit-and-research-projects/each-baby-counts-learn-support/escalation-toolkit/teach-or-treat

29. Trowler P. Higher Education Policy and Institution Change: Intentions and Outcomes in Turbulent Environments [e-book]. Available from: https://read.amazon.co.uk/?asin=B006W0G3HQ

30. Khan A. Policy implementation, some aspects and issues. J Community Posit Pract. 2016;16(3):3–12. Available from: https://www.researchgate.net/publication/320549262_POLICY_IMPLEMENTATION_SOME_ASPECTS_AND_ISSUES

31. Ball S, Maguire M, Braun A. How schools do policy: policy enactments in secondary schools [Internet]. Available from: https://www.researchgate.net/publication/288772450_How_Schools_Do_Policy_Policy_Enactments_in_Secondary_Schools

32. Bardach E, Patashnik E. A practical guide for policy analysis: the eightfold path to more effective problem solving. 6th ed. Washington, DC: QC Press; 2019.

33. Steer R, Spours A, Hodgson I, Finlay F, Coffield S, Edward S, Gregson M. Modernisation and the role of policy levers in the learning and skills sector. J Vocat Educ Train. 2007;59(2):175–92.

34. Hyatt D. The critical policy discourse analysis frame: helping doctoral students engage with the educational policy analysis. Teach High Educ. 2013;18(8):833–45. https://doi.org/10.1080/13562517.2013.795935.

35. The Lancet. Lancet. 2021;398(10306):1105–94. Available from: https://www.thelancet.com/journals/lancet/issue/vol398no10306/PIIS0140-6736(21)X0040-2

36. Horton R. A statement from the Editor-in-Chief on The Lancet cover quote [Internet]. London: The Lancet; 2021. Available from: https://www.thelancet.com/

37. Fairclough N. Analysing discourse and text: textual analysis for social research. London: Routledge; 2003.

38. Independent review of maternity services at Shrewsbury and Telford Hospital NHS Trust. Ockenden Report: findings, conclusions and essential actions. London: GOV.UK; 2022. Available from: https://www.gov.uk/government/publications/final-report-of-the-ockenden-review

39. Independent Investigation into East Kent Maternity Services. Maternity and neonatal services in East Kent – the Report of the Independent Investigation. London: GOV.UK; 2022. Available from: https://www.gov.uk/government/publications/maternity-and-neonatal-services-in-east-kent-reading-the-signals-report

40. Haddon C. The Nimrod Review: an independent review into the broader issues surrounding the loss of the RAF Nimrod MR2 aircraft XV230 in Afghanistan in 2006 [Internet]. London: The Stationery Office; 2009. Available from: https://www.gov.uk/government/publications/the-nimrod-review

41. Magyari-Beck I. Identifying blocks to creativity in Hungarian culture. Creat Res J. 1991;4:419–27.

42. Cremin T, Chappell K. Creative pedagogies: a systematic review. Res Pap Educ. 2019;36:1–33. https://doi.org/10.1080/02671522.2019.1677757.

43. Gardiner P. Playwriting and flow: the interconnection between creativity, engagement and skill development. Int J Educ Arts. 2017:18.

44. Gardiner P, Anderson M. Structured creative processes in learning playwriting: invoking imaginative pedagogies. Camb J Educ. 2018;48:1–20. https://doi.org/10.1080/0305764X.2016.1267710.

45. Andina-Díaz E, et al. Lack of autonomy and professional recognition as major factors for burnout in midwives: a systematic mixed-method review. J Adv Nurs [Preprint]. 2024; https://doi.org/10.1111/jan.16279.

46. Maslach C, Jackson SE, Leiter MP. Maslach Burnout inventory. Lanham: Scarecrow Education; 1997.

47. Li CP, He LP. Trait creativity among midwifery students: a cross-sectional study. Rev Assoc Med Bras (1992). 2023;69(4):e20221355. doi:https://doi.org/10.1590/1806-9282.20221355. PMID: 37075447; PMCID: PMC10176656.

Positive Workplace Culture Principles and Ways Forward

6

Introduction

This chapter draws together key principles from prior chapters to demarcate clear strategies and principles that contribute towards creating a positive workplace culture. The chapter highlights what is understood in current evidence and where further research is needed. You are encouraged to create vision, plan and take practical steps forward to contribute at the individual level towards building a positive workplace culture. The chapter is organised under four subheadings, each providing focus on the ways forward by the following:

1. Practising and participating in ways that build positive social and interpersonal skills
2. Leading to support wellbeing with compassion and sociocultural awareness
3. Engaging with team idea-sharing, ownership and learning
4. Taking and giving opportunities for individual, group and system learning

The chapter focusses on making sense of and understanding the strengths and limitations of social and culture-based practice principles in your workplace. Conflicts or challenges in action and change are explored further to aid you in drawing connections between self and culture, to develop your individual workplace resilience as part of the process of change and to understand the complexities of workplace culture change. Closure is achieved by revisiting realistic and meaningful understanding about how you can contribute towards culture change while also recognising and overcoming factors of counterinfluence and challenge.

© The Author(s), under exclusive license to Springer Nature Switzerland AG 2025
L. Philp-von Woyna, *Unravelling Workplace Culture in Healthcare*,
https://doi.org/10.1007/978-3-032-11771-7_6

Individual, Interpersonal and Social-Based Principles that Build a Positive Workplace Culture

Individual, interpersonal and social-based principles that build a positive culture relate to exploring how you behave in the social context as contributing towards workplace culture. This understanding is grounded in theoretical understanding called *social constructivism* [1]. This understanding suggests that the social behaviours of individuals and the behaviours of those as groups build and construct realities, including the workplace culture. This understanding suggests that the behaviour of individuals really does matter because it actively builds the group culture. While this perspective receives some criticism because it is limited in consideration of some influences such as issues of power and policy, it offers valuable insight and understanding about how individual and social-based skills and action can feed into wider issues. In this section, issues of individual agency (action), and more specific workplace behaviours, such as gossip and unprofessional behaviour are explored as *constructing* the wider workplace culture.

Practicing Individual Agency *Actively Builds* Workplace Culture

A positive workplace culture can be cultivated, but it relies on individuals practicing in ways that support positive group principles [2]. Every workplace collectively cultivates certain behaviours and practices that become acceptable within the group, and individuals play an *active* role in approving, praising and valuing certain behaviours/actions and in disapproving of other behaviours/actions. Through individual *action or inaction*, different types of social behaviour can be fostered, encouraged or shut down (stopped) by individuals [2, 3]. Past experiences within group cultures shape future participation. For instance, if ideas were previously dismissed, individuals may hesitate to contribute again [4], but individual contributions, even small ones, can drive critical improvements [5]. Overcoming the fear and hesitation you may experience to motivate yourself to make contributions at work might provide those vital contributions that make a difference. Literature suggests that we are motivated to act and share ideas by both intrinsic factors, such as personal fulfilment, passion and self-expression and extrinsic factors like recognition or rewards [6]. The intrinsically motivating factors are considered *vital* for psychological well-being and self-actualisation according to humanistic theory [7]. Therefore, environments that support individual expression and active engagement by individuals through opportunities that enable the surfacing of personal fulfilment, passion for topics and self-expression can enhance individual mental health, job satisfaction and resilience, making it a key consideration in workplace culture change and development.

Reflective Point
How can you engage with sharing your opinion, ideas or questions surrounding an
   issue that is personally meaningful to you, or you are passionate about?

Participate in Workplace Gossip

Workplace gossip is an expected social behaviour in healthcare [8]. Gossip is
defined as verbal evaluative communication among individuals about another person who is usually not present. It means the topic of gossip might be either positively affirming or negative, but it is an expected, everyday aspect of conversation
because evaluating others (making judgements of people and how people act in situations) often forms the basis of communicating information to one another. Positive
gossip in the workplace can be a powerful means of expressing what is valued and
what behaviours you believe should be cultivated, whereas negative gossip can be a
warning sign of organisational dysfunction and failure [9]. It can also uncover areas
of risk and concern from colleagues that have not been raised formally. Box 6.1
summarises analysis of workplace gossip and what this could indicate.

Box 6.1 Interpreting Gossip Topics to Identify Workplace Challenges
- Gossip focussed on senior colleagues may indicate power imbalance or
   leadership issues.
- Gossip focussed on junior colleagues may reflect unclear expectations,
   communication with those colleagues or (power-based) bullying.
- Uncertainty about aspects of communication suggests trust and hierarchy
   problems.
- Work task-related gossip may point to burnout, poor support or unclear roles.
- Gossip about a person's characteristics is bullying and must be addressed
   directly.
- Gossip for *a sense of belonging* reflects low trust and poor team cohesion.
- Organisational change-related gossip signals poor leadership and commu-
   nication about change or individuals processing change.
- Power-enhancing gossip (for the gossiper) may indicate dominant leader-
   ship issues or bullying.

Negative gossip in the workplace often signals deeper cultural issues such as
poor communication, power imbalances, lack of trust and unclear roles [10]. The
nature of gossip, whether focused on leadership, junior staff, tasks or personal matters, can reveal specific organisational challenges (see Box 1.2). Addressing these
issues requires strategies like improving leadership, clarifying expectations, fostering trust and tackling bullying. Individual health workers can make a difference
contributing towards addressing many of these issues. This is because individuals

engage in gossip and social interaction in the workplace on a daily basis meaning your communication (through action or inaction) can either support (cultivate) or shut down (abandon) different social behaviours. Ultimately, the type of gossip you engage with and social behaviours you participate in shape the workplace culture. Recognition of social behaviours and how you contribute to different behaviours can aid in creating safer, more inclusive workplace culture.

Reflective Point
How do you talk about other people in the workplace? Do you engage in positive or negative gossip and how do you think this is contributing to the workplace culture?

Respond to Bullying and Unprofessional Behaviour

Social cliques and bullying in the workplace often stem from a desire for belonging but can lead to exclusion, gossip and unsafe working environments. These behaviours undermine teamwork and psychological safety, especially in high-pressure settings like healthcare [5]. Addressing bullying requires collective responsibility not just individual action but support from peers, leaders, organisations and wider systems [11]. Effective strategies include respectfully naming and challenging unprofessional behaviour, using compassionate approaches (where appropriate) and considering the power dynamics of behaviours [12]. Documentation of incidents, rather than gossiping with those involved, is essential for clarity and accountability and supporting victims through small but meaningful actions, such as validating concerns or helping escalate issues can collectively shift workplace culture.

Individuals can take steps to support others and shut down problem behaviour by actively standing by colleagues, seeking support when needed and taking thoughtful steps to challenge inappropriate conduct. When individuals encounter unprofessional behaviour or bullying, it can be helpful to reflect on the broader impact of it and share your thoughts in escalating concerns. For instance, you may consider how the behaviour affects autonomy and reflects systemic issues and how it can shape future learning and problematic behaviour. Clear and collective learning from problematic behaviours can help to prevent recurrence. This requires action from compassionate leaders [13], but also the actions and response of all within the team. For example, at an individual level, strategies such as respectfully naming behaviours and using compassionate, supportive language can help create a psychologically safer, more inclusive environment.

Ultimately, building a respectful, psychologically safe workplace depends on recognising the impact of social behaviours and promoting *collective action* to address bullying and unprofessional behaviour. These efforts are vital for creating a culture of safety, trust and wellbeing in healthcare settings.

Reflective Point
How can you participate in *collective action* that addresses unprofessional behaviour in the workplace?

Leadership that Supports a Positive Workplace Culture

Leadership in healthcare is incredibly important for cultivating a positive workplace culture. Strong, positive leaders set clear boundaries and expectations, advocate for staff, build trust with colleagues, promote team cohesion and create stability while working towards a clear vision and during times of organisational change. Leaders can create psychologically safe environments where individuals feel empowered to raise concerns, ask questions, share ideas and prioritise person-centred care [14]. Leadership can actively take steps to encourage open communication and support a learning culture and collective ownership of problems and problem-solving. Leaders can prioritise and influence a learning culture by practising in ways that consider the group sociocultural context and opportunities for learning and change. Key influential factors that are largely influenced by leaders and include the local processes that people are exposed to that encourage idea generation, the prompting of idea-sharing through local opportunity and whether the acceptability and readiness to receive new ideas [15]. Essentially, whether change and innovation begins depends on all the sociocultural factors, of which leaders are largely influential. The right environmental climate is needed to accept new ideas, people need cognitive skills to generate ideas, processes that encourage idea development and practical prompts, support and examples of ideas to grow personally and professionally. This section covers compassionate leadership, leadership that promotes idea-sharing and organisation-level actions that contribute towards building a positive workplace culture.

Healthcare Needs Compassionate Leaders

Compassionate leadership is increasingly recognised as essential for fostering safe, inclusive and high-performing healthcare environments [14]. It involves intentional listening, understanding diverse perspectives, empathising with others and taking meaningful action to support staff [13, 16]. This approach shifts workplace culture away from blame and punishment, towards learning and psychological safety [16].

Compassion itself is multidimensional, encompassing compassion for others, from others, and self-compassion which is interconnected with individual wellbeing [17]. Compassionate leadership plays a critical role in shaping whether individuals feel confident and safe to speak up and contribute solutions, opinions or ideas [18]. Every healthcare worker needs to understand how they can expect a compassionate leader or manager to behave which includes attitudes and behaviours of openness, empathy and responsive action to ensure individual wellbeing and enable effective, safe work. Individual-level expectations of leadership play a role in holding leaders accountable, but support is needed from an organisational and regulatory perspective as well. Regulatory bodies like the Nursing and Midwifery Council (NMC) [14] and the Royal College of Obstetricians and Gynaecologists (RCOG) [19] advocate for compassionate leadership as a foundation for safe, high-quality care. However, individuals also require understanding to appreciate that local leadership alone is not enough; organisational support, national professional and policy frameworks also need to reinforce these values to ensure accountability and drive cultural change. Ultimately, collective action is essential to embed compassion into everyday practice and leadership to support a positive and learning culture.

Reflective Point

How can you ensure you are practising compassionately through intentional listening, understanding diverse perspectives, empathising with others and taking meaningful action to support others?

Organisations and Leaders Need to Prioritise Staff Wellbeing

Organisation-level and local-level leadership and management is critical to support the wellbeing of individual staff and to foster a positive and learning culture. This is beneficial for both staff and patients because one of the biggest challenges in healthcare relates to the wellbeing of staff [20]. Pressure on staff working in the UK health system is increasing as a combination of staff shortages, resource constriction, limited finances, high turnover of staff and increasing workloads collides [20]. This is increasing the number of errors, adversely impacting healthcare workers wellbeing and reducing patient safety [21]. Organisations need to support a range practices and priorities that promote the wellbeing of staff. These can be summarised under four key actionable areas, namely:

1. Meeting the basic needs of people at work
2. Promoting a learning culture
3. Group problem-ownership and problem-solving
4. Supporting individual development

Combined these priorities can support a positive, learning culture from an organisational level. Each area is summarised as follows:

1. *Meeting the basic needs of people* can include supporting practices such as flexible working. In 2025, the Working Families Index identified healthcare as the UK's most inflexible employing industry [22], with sectors like marketing, banking, and education offering more flexible options. Flexible working, defined as greater choice in when, where and how work is done, supports wellbeing, reduces stress and improves retention and patient safety [23, 24]

   Despite these benefits, the British Medical Journal (BMJ) highlighted the NHS's institutional resistance to flexibility [25]. At a 2023 roundtable, experts including Rachel Hutchings (Nuffield Trust, Future Proof report) and Dr. Farzana

Hussain (GP) discussed how negative workplace culture and fear of stigma deter staff from requesting flexible arrangements. The BMJ proposed six strategies to improve flexibility [25]:

- Proactive support—Employers should actively promote flexible options.
- Learning from primary care—Adjusting service times to support staff needs.
- Better planning—Flexibility requires strategic workforce planning, not fear.
- Role modelling—Senior staff working flexibly can shift expectations and culture.
- Embrace the challenge—Adapting services collaboratively is possible.
- Patient involvement—Patients should help shape realistic care models.

To attract and retain healthcare workers, workplaces must offer decent conditions and fair pay and protect worker rights. This includes meeting basic needs such as access to rest areas, food, water and facilities for breastfeeding, alongside time for rest and hydration. Reports show that even these basic needs are often unmet in healthcare settings [26], increasing the risk of errors and compromising patient safety.

2. *Promoting a learning culture* requires organisational support, especially surrounding investigation of errors and incidents. While errors are inevitable in complex systems, they often reveal systemic flaws rather than individual failings. However, a persistent blame culture in healthcare places undue responsibility on individuals, causing psychological harm. A tragic example involved a nurse who died by suicide following a system failure and fear of blame [27], and the General Medical Council found at least 28 suicides linked to fitness-to-practice investigations, highlighting the damaging impact of blame cultures. To address this, NHS England introduced the Patient Safety Incident Response Framework (PSIRF) [28], promoting principles such as focussing on learning rather than investigation processes, avoiding individual blame to uncover systemic issues, encouraging collaboration and psychological safety and supporting open dialogue and curiosity from leadership. Fear of retribution discourages transparency, underscoring the need for team-based learning and problem-solving approaches.

3. *Group problem-solving* is a vital yet often overlooked component of fostering a learning culture in healthcare [18]. Effective team-based improvement depends on shared ownership of challenges, supported by strong interpersonal relationships and a culture that encourages transparency and collaboration. When errors are treated as group problems rooted in systemic issues, rather than individual failings, psychological safety, wellbeing and better solutions emerge [18]. Promoting group ownership involves open communication about errors, candid discussions focussed on prevention and prioritising learning over blame. Success depends not only on team dynamics but also on local workplace politics and broader social and economic contexts. Recognising that individuals operate within larger systems helps explain why cultural change can be difficult, yet possible. When individuals contribute ideas and engage with team dynamics, they shape group functioning and enhance emotional wellbeing. Sharing ideas is a

key developmental milestone for professional growth, and in healthcare, this involves navigating complex social and professional environments to aid group learning [18]. To support this, staff need opportunities to understand workplace norms and feel safe expressing their perspectives. This fosters innovation, strengthens learning cultures and improves patient safety and care quality [29].

4. *Supporting individual development* in healthcare is essential not only for personal growth but also for strengthening teams and organisations [18]. Opportunities to understand workplace culture, challenges and strengths help staff share ideas and drive improvements. Since organisational culture reflects the *collective values* of its people, investing in individuals directly benefits the wider system. Despite evidence that education and development improve safety and retention [30], investment beyond initial training remains limited restricting career progression and job satisfaction. The NHS Long-Term Workforce Plan aims to address these issues by increasing training places, improving wellbeing and reforming care delivery [31]. To support staff development, strategies must include recognition and reward, such as career progression and fair remuneration. Ultimately, investing in individual development is a strategic move to enhance workforce wellbeing, retention and healthcare quality.

Reflective Point
What action can you take to promote wellbeing practice at work?

Changing Workplace Culture as a Team

Workplace behaviour is shaped by normative roles and mindsets. Hierarchies influence communication, decision-making and safety and are reinforced through workplace culture and socialisation [18]. Roles and authority are socially constructed and can be challenged to improve collaboration and care.

Sociocultural theory emphasises the sociocultural foundations of behaviours such as learning, creativity and culture change [34]. It highlights the interdependence between individuals and their social, material and psychological environments. Sociocultural perspectives explain how behaviour is shaped by living in a socially connected and materially embedded world [34]. It means that efforts to change embedded culture in healthcare need to consider the context of the culture. There are social aspects, psychological aspects and material (physical and role/power-based issues) that require attention and collaborative solutions.

Learning Culture Is a Team Issue and *Critical* for Culture Change

A stagnant workplace culture in healthcare can hinder growth, innovation and staff engagement, often leading to high turnover, poor communication and low morale. Individuals in such environments may resist change and adhere to outdated practices, limiting motivation to improve or adapt. In contrast, a learning culture promotes continuous improvement, autonomy and adaptability, supporting staff in acquiring new skills and solving problems to enhance care. Understanding workplace culture as both individual and socially enacted is essential, particularly in recognising how professionals are *socialised* into existing norms through their desire for acceptance and belonging. This *socialisation* process, explained by Social Learning Theory [32], can reinforce either positive or problematic behaviours depending on the dominant culture [33]. To foster meaningful change, individuals should reflect on their own beliefs about workplace norms and explore culture-based diversity within teams. Exposure to different team cultures and professional roles can improve collaboration and care quality. Tools like the Competing Values Framework (CVF) [33] can help individuals assess dominant cultural traits, offering insights into whether a team is more flexible or stable and whether it prioritises internal wellbeing or external performance. This can aid perspectival dialogue, which involves engaging with varied viewpoints, ideas and collaborative learning [34]. Movement involving networking and working across teams, departments and organisations can support new understanding and learning. Exposure to different experiences and information can challenge existing assumptions, creating dissonance that promotes growth and collective problem-solving. In contrast, isolated teams are less equipped for change, and it can restrict group learning. Those that expand their networks, locally and globally, are better positioned to innovate and adapt [18].

Understanding global diversity in perspectives can significantly enrich idea-sharing and foster a more inclusive learning culture. Perceptions and professional interactions are shaped not only by workplace dynamics but also by broader social and cultural contexts specific to the country where we live and our understanding, which influence how we approach problems and collaborate. Learning can emerge from interconnected systems, including environments, relationships, policies and processes that span cultural boundaries. These diverse ecologies enable a wide range of creative expressions and problem-solving approaches. Ideas and understanding can also come from cross-industry learning. For example, the Nimrod Review called for a fundamental shift in safety culture within the Ministry of Defence and the armed forces, emphasising the need for *proactive safety* practices and *open reporting without fear of reprisal.* Drawing on best practices from civil aviation, the review advocated for a *principle-based approach to safety,* prioritising learning, collaboration, and *system integrity* over rigid rule-following and hierarchical control. This can bring a new perspective to challenges within healthcare that can lead to better solutions.

Reflective Point

How can you personally contribute towards supporting a group learning culture?

How can you gain a wider range of perspectives on workplace issues?

Everyday Conversations in Healthcare Teams Matter

Organisational culture is deeply reflected in everyday conversations, which shapes relationships, wellbeing and collective problem-solving. In healthcare, the quality of dialogue between colleagues influences not only individual psychological wellbeing but also team purpose and the development of ideas and learning. While ideas often begin with individuals, their growth and implementation depend on the surrounding social-professional network [35]. The theory of the 'network of enterprise' highlights how ideas evolve through interaction within systems and social contexts [35]. While fear of rejection and entrenched group norms can inhibit idea-sharing, especially in environments resistant to change, historical examples, such as Darwin's hesitancy to share his theories, illustrate how *social dynamics* can both hinder and enable innovation [35]. Encouraging open, constructive conversations and recognising the influence of group culture on personal apprehension can help overcome these barriers, fostering a more inclusive, creative and wellbeing-focussed workplace. Improving workplace dialogue and the sharing of questions, opinions, critical thoughts, ideas and solutions is essential for fostering a positive team culture, enhancing wellbeing and supporting collaborative problem-solving [18].

Strategies for promoting team dialogue that can build positive workplace culture include creating informal spaces for every day, meaningful conversation, as follows:

1. *Conversational approaches* such as the 'cup of coffee' approach that encourages non-judgmental peer dialogue around concerning behaviours [19].
2. *Moving beyond active listening* by recognising layers of communication among team members that reflect facts, values, and emotions which can deepen understanding during conflict (see Box 4.4).
3. *Being curious and open* in questioning to help uncover root causes of tension among teams, while balancing challenge with support fostering trust and openness.
4. *Honest, constructive conversations* that give feedback while prioritising mutual understanding that can strengthen relationships and promote learning.
5. *Making conservations purposeful* by agreeing on clear actions and shared accountability. Clarity in conversation can ensure conversations lead to meaningful change empowering individuals to contribute to a healthier workplace culture.

How we communicate with each other on a daily basis at work can serve to promote positive workplace culture principles.

Reflective Point
How can you ensure that everyday conservations promote a positive workplace culture?

Opportunities in Education and Policy to Change Workplace Culture

Engage in Sociocultural Education Opportunities

Workplace culture education is essential for driving meaningful change in healthcare. Awareness of acceptable and unacceptable behaviours should be embedded in every healthcare professional's education, yet it remains absent from mandatory UK undergraduate training [18]. Even regulatory bodies face cultural challenges with the Nursing and Midwifery Council [36] recently identifying internal issues including discrimination, low trust, micromanagement and lack of accountability. In response, the NMC outlined five focus areas for culture change: leadership capability, psychological safety and inclusion, accountability, learning and multi-professional collaboration. Embedding understanding of these principles and other sociocultural principles that influence workplace culture could be beneficial to changing workplace culture through improving awareness and skills for those entering health professions. Education surrounding these issues matters because supportive workplace cultures lead to better patient outcomes, improved decision making and improved staff wellbeing [37]. Educational leadership as well as clinical leadership is central to shaping culture, influencing staff and student health professional confidence, care quality and culture learning.

Educator preparation is currently underfunded and inconsistent. There are no formal requirements for clinical supervisors to be trained in workplace culture or sociocultural factors and formal education qualifications for teachers are reducing. For instance, the proportion of midwifery educators with master's-level qualifications has dropped from 70% in 2018 to 40% in 2023, and only 10% hold doctorates [38]. Education empowers individuals to think critically, solve problems and influence policy and practice. Students are highly sensitive to senior approval [18], reflecting a desire for legitimacy within the profession that shapes their behaviour and socialisation to culture-based norms [32]. This means it is imperative to invest in education that builds confidence and provides thinking and practical tools for change enabling staff to challenge poor practices and contribute to culture transformation [18]. Social movement and educational theory highlights how individuals can understand power dynamics within hierarchical structures that unintentionally reinforce problems. Education is essential to inform challenging of these influences through open dialogue and inclusive practices. Diversity in educational experiences and creative pedagogical practices in healthcare education can help individuals to experience the problems from different physical or social positions that better inform collaborative solutions. Ultimately, culture change is most effective when individuals have the knowledge and skills to reflect, collaborate and act across all levels of the system.

Reflective Point
What steps can you take to engage in diverse educational experiences to enrich your
understanding and ideas to solve culture-based problems?

Local Policy and Micro-politics Within Teams

Policy acts as a powerful tool for driving change in healthcare, shaped by complex
social, political, economic and cultural factors [39]. Its development is influenced
by national, local and global forces, including supranational agents and popular
trends [40]. Theories such as pluralism and elitism offer contrasting views on how
policy is formed, either through broad stakeholder input or by a select few and regulatory bodies also play a role in *legitimising* policy through formal procedures.
Despite theories, the case of Martha Mills exemplifies how individual experiences
can shape national policy. Following her preventable death from sepsis, Martha's
Rule was introduced to ensure patients and families can raise concerns and request
second opinions, highlighting the importance of agency and advocacy of individuals in policy formation [41]. This case underscores how reflective learning from
specific incidents can inform broader health policy and how healthcare professionals and individuals alike contribute to shaping policy through feedback, action and
leadership.

Policy implementation is often debated as either a distinct phase or an integral
part of the broader policy-making process. While some view it as a goal-oriented
sequence of actions, others argue it is a dynamic process shaped by institutional
contexts and discourses. Critical analysis of policy helps uncover its drivers, whether
stemming from deficits or excesses and reveals how sociopolitical values influence
its formation and enactment. This can help individuals understand how policy contributes towards local, enacted behaviours and decisions and subsequently workplace culture. Analysing policy and policy language and context can expose
competing influences and guide improvements in both policy creation and
implementation.

The enactment of policy is also influenced by micro-politics. Micro-politics
refers to everyday power dynamics within healthcare settings, such as how shift
leaders or senior staff use their authority to shape team decisions and relationships.
These dynamics can either foster or suppress innovation, particularly when power is
misused to restrict autonomy or favour certain individuals [18]. Local workplace
culture and micro-politics significantly influence whether healthcare improvement
ideas were shared and supported in my doctoral research [18]. The study found that
broader political issues, such as national maternity safety investigations, motivated
staff to generate ideas for change, including addressing racial inequalities and promoting culturally sensitive care. However, local micro-political factors often constrained these ideas, especially when senior staff dismissed suggestions due to
resource limitations or entrenched norms. For example, a student's proposal to
extend postnatal care was rejected due to local policy and lack of support from
experienced midwives. This illustrates how both local and national politics shape

healthcare improvement efforts. The study aligns with wider literature showing that experienced professionals play a key role in enabling or hindering innovation. It suggests that interventions encouraging senior staff to collaborate with junior colleagues while remaining open to new ideas could enhance learning cultures and drive meaningful change.

Reflective Point
How can you participate in the local formation of policy? How can you change
   workplace culture at the micro-political level?

Summary

This final chapter has revisited some of the core aspects of the book. Here you have had opportunity to reflect on ways forward and how you can contribute towards changing healthcare culture through individual agency. Culture-based problems are often unique to the specific context and group of people, but because culture is built and sustained locally, solutions and change can emerge from local collaborative efforts.

By focussing on the four key areas of this chapter, I hope that you feel empowered to practice positive interpersonal and social skills, engage in meaningful conversations with colleagues, challenge unprofessional and bullying behaviour in effective, collaborative ways, lead with compassion and wellbeing in mind, support a learning culture, participate in policy development and engage with educational opportunities to diversify your understanding and improve personal-professional development.

References

1. Arthur J, Waring M, Coe R, Hedges L, editors. Research methods and methodologies in education. London: SAGE; 2012.
2. Smith T. Plato and education [Internet]. EBSCO; 2021. Available from: https://www.ebsco.com/research-starters/education/plato-and-education.
3. Anderson C, Cropley A. Correlates of originality. Aust J Psychiatry. 1966;18(1):218–27.
4. Wormington S. Better culture starts with compassionate leadership [Internet]. Center for Creative Leadership; 2024. Available from: https://www.ccl.org/articles/better-culture-starts-with-compassionate-leadership.
5. Edmondson A. The fearless organization: creating psychological safety in the workplace for learning, innovation, and growth. Hoboken: Wiley; 2018.
6. Hanchett Hanson M, Amato A, Durani A, Hoyden J, Koe S, Sheagren E, Yang Y. Creativity and improvised educations: case studies for understanding impact and implications. London: Routledge; 2021.
7. Maslow A. The farther reaches of human nature. New York: Viking; 1971.
8. Georganta K, Panagopoulou E, Montgomery A. Talking behind their backs: negative gossip and burnout in hospitals [Internet]. 2014. Available from: https://doi.org/10.1016/j.burn.2014.07.003

9. Oliver C. Reflexive inquiry and the strange loop tool. Hum Syst. 2004;15(2):127–40. Available from: https://cmminstitute.org/wp-content/uploads/2020/12/Human-Systems-2004-Oliver.pdf.

10. Michelson G, van Iterson A, Waddington K. Gossip in organizations: contexts, consequences, and controversies. Group Organ Manag. 2010;35(4):371–90. https://doi.org/10.1177/1059601109360389.

11. Gaffney H, Ttofi MM, Farrington DP. What works in anti-bullying programs? Analysis of effective intervention components. J Sch Psychol. 2021;85:37–56. https://doi.org/10.1016/j.jsp.2020.12.002. PMID: 33715780.

12. Royal College of Obstetricians and Gynaecologists. Improving workplace behaviours: workplace behaviour toolkit [Internet]. London: RCOG; 2021. Available from: https://www.rcog.org.uk/careers-and-training/workforce/improving-workplace-behaviours/workplace-behaviour-toolkit/.

13. Bailey S, West M. What is compassionate leadership? [Internet]. London: The King's Fund; 2022. Available from: https://www.kingsfund.org.uk/publications/what-is-compassionate-leadership.

14. Nursing and Midwifery Council. Supporting nursing and midwifery leaders to ensure the best possible care [Internet]. London: NMC; 2023. Available from: https://www.nmc.org.uk/news/news-and-updates/supporting-nursing-and-midwifery-leaders-to-ensure-the-best-possible-care.

15. Cremin T, Chappell K. Creative pedagogies: a systematic review. Res Pap Educ. 2019;36:1–33. https://doi.org/10.1080/02671522.2019.1677757.

16. Edmondson AC, Lei Z. Psychological safety: the history, renaissance, and future of an interpersonal construct [Internet]. 2014. Available from: https://doi.org/10.1146/annurev-orgpsych-031413-091305.

17. Gilbert P, Catarino F, Duarte C, et al. The development of compassionate engagement and action scales for self and others. J Compassionate Health Care. 2017;4:4. https://doi.org/10.1186/s40639-017-0033-3.

18. Philp-Von Woyna L. A multi-case study to understand the ways in which sociocultural factors influence everyday creative contributions in healthcare and higher education by student midwives. Doctoral thesis. Staffordshire: Staffordshire University; 2025. Available from: https://eprints.staffs.ac.uk/8884/.

19. Royal College of Obstetricians and Gynaecologists. Teach or treat [Internet]. London: RCOG; n.d. Available from: https://www.rcog.org.uk/about-us/quality-improvement-clinical-audit-and-research-projects/each-baby-counts-learn-support/escalation-toolkit/teach-or-treat.

20. Dunn P, Ewbank L, Alderwick H. Nine major challenges facing health and care in England. London: The Health Foundation; 2023. Available from: https://www.health.org.uk/reports-and-analysis/briefings/nine-major-challenges-facing-health-and-care-in-england.

21. Brennan PA, Oeppen RS. The role of human factors in improving patient safety. Trends Urol Mens Health. 2022;13(3):30–3. https://doi.org/10.1002/tre.858.

22. Working Families. Working Families Index 2025: employer briefing [Internet]. London: Working Families; 2025. Available from: https://workingfamilies.org.uk.

23. Ray TK, Pana-Cryan R. Work flexibility and work-related Well-being. Int J Environ Res Public Health. 2021;18(6):3254. https://doi.org/10.3390/ijerph18063254.

24. Halpern DF. How time-flexible work policies can reduce stress, improve health, and save money. Stress Health. 2005;21(3):157–68. https://doi.org/10.1002/smi.1049.

25. Lacobucci G. Improving flexible working in the NHS. BMJ. 2023;380:618. https://doi.org/10.1136/bmj.p618.

26. Castella T. Banning drinking water for staff on wards "misguided", warns union. Nurs Times. 2021. Available from: https://www.nursingtimes.net.

27. Radhakrishna S. Culture of blame in the National Health Service; consequences and solutions. Br J Anaesth. 2015;115(5):653–5. Available from: https://www.bjanaesthesia.org.

28. NHS England. Patient safety incident response framework: oversight roles and responsibilities specification. Version 1 [Internet]. London: NHS England; 2022. Available from: https://www.england.nhs.uk/publication/patient-safety-incident-response-framework-supporting-guidance.

29. Andina-Díaz E, et al. Lack of autonomy and professional recognition as major factors for burnout in midwives: a systematic mixed-method review. J Adv Nurs [Preprint]. 2024. https://doi.org/10.1111/jan.16279.

30. NHS England. NHS health and wellbeing strategic overview [Internet]. London: NHS England; 2022. Available from: https://www.england.nhs.uk/publication/nhs-health-and-wellbeing-framework.

31. NHS England. NHS long term workforce plan [Internet]. London: NHS England; 2023. Available from: https://www.england.nhs.uk/publication/nhs-long-term-workforce-plan.

32. Lave J, Wenger E. Situated learning: legitimate peripheral participation. Cambridge: Cambridge University Press; 1991.

33. Quinn R, Rohrbaugh J. A spatial model of effectiveness criteria: toward a competing values approach to organizational analysis. Manag Sci. 1983;29:363–77. https://doi.org/10.1287/mnsc.29.3.363.

34. Glăveanu VP. A sociocultural theory of creativity: bridging the social, the material and the psychological. Rev Gen Psychol. 2020;24(4):335–54.

35. Wallace DB, Gruber HE. The case study method and evolving systems approach for understanding unique creative people at work. In: Sternberg RJ, editor. Handbook of creativity. Cambridge: Cambridge University Press; 1999.

36. Nursing and Midwifery Council. Culture transformation plan 2025–2028 [pdf]. London: NMC; 2025. Available from: https://www.nmc.org.uk/globalassets/sitedocuments/independent-reviews/2025/nmc-culture-transformation-plan-2025.pdf.

37. West THR, Daher P, Dawson JF, Lyubovnikova J, Buttigieg SC, West MA. The relationship between leader support, staff influence over decision making, work pressure and patient satisfaction: a cross-sectional analysis of NHS datasets in England. BMJ Open. 2022. https://doi.org/10.1136/bmjopen-2021-052778.

38. Royal College of Midwives. State of midwifery education 2023 [pdf]. London: RCM; 2023. Available from: https://www.rcm.org.uk/publications/state-of-midwifery-education-2023/.

39. Forrester G, Garratt D. Education policy unravelled. 2nd ed. London: Bloomsbury; 2016.

40. Ball S. The education debate. 2nd ed. Bristol: Policy Press; 2013.

41. NHS England. Implementation of first phase of Martha's rule [Internet]. London: NHS England; 2024. Available from: https://www.england.nhs.uk/.

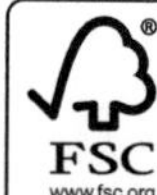

MIX
Papier aus verantwortungsvollen Quellen
Paper from responsible sources
FSC® C105338

If you have any concerns about our products,
you can contact us on
ProductSafety@springernature.com

In case Publisher is established outside the EU,
the EU authorized representative is:
Springer Nature Customer Service Center GmbH
Europaplatz 3, 69115 Heidelberg, Germany

Printed by Libri Plureos GmbH
in Hamburg, Germany